A GUIDE TO

cancer genetics in

CLINICAL PRACTICE

Edited by Sue Clark

tfm Publishing Limited, Castle Hill Barns, Harley, Nr Shrewsbury, SY5 6LX, UK. Tel: +44 (0)1952 510061; Fax: +44 (0)1952 510192 E-mail: nikki@tfmpublishing.com; Web site: www.tfmpublishing.com

Design & Typesetting: Nikki Bramhill BSc Hons Dip Law
First Edition: © May 2009
Front cover image: © Comstock Inc., www.comstock.com

ISBN: 978 1 903378 54 0

Printed by Gutenberg Press Ltd., Gudja Road, Tarxien, PLA 19, Malta. Tel: +356 21897037; Fax: +356 21800069.

Contents

Contributors

Andrew Beggs MRCS Research Registrar in Colorectal Surgery, Mayday University Hospital, London, and Honorary Research Fellow in Cancer Genetics, St George's, University of London, UK

Vanessa Blair BHB MBChB Surgical Research Fellow, Department of Surgery, University of Auckland, Auckland, New Zealand

John Burn MD FRCP FRCPCH FRCOG FMedSci Professor of Clinical Genetics, Newcastle University, Newcastle upon Tyne, UK

Sue Clark MD FRCS (Gen Surg) Consultant Colorectal Surgeon and Assistant Director, The Polyposis Registry, St Mark's Hospital, Harrow, UK

Charis Eng MD PhD FACP Sondra J and Stephen R Hardis Chair of Cancer Genomic Medicine; Chairman and Director, Genomic Medicine Institute; Director, Center for Personalized Genetic Healthcare, Lerner Research Institute, Cleveland Clinic, Cleveland, Ohio, USA; Professor and Vice Chairman of Genetics, Case Western Reserve University School of Medicine, Cleveland, Ohio, USA

Brandie Heald MS CGC Certified Genetic Counselor, Center for Personalized Genetic Healthcare, Lerner Research Institute, Cleveland Clinic, Cleveland, Ohio, USA

Shirley Hodgson FRCP DM Professor of Cancer Genetics, St George's, University of London, and Honorary Consultant, St George's Hospital, London, UK

Matthew F Kalady MD Staff Surgeon, Department of Colorectal Surgery, Digestive Disease Institute, Cleveland Clinic, Cleveland, Ohio, USA

Fiona Lalloo MD FRCP Consultant in Clinical Genetics, St Mary's Hospital, Manchester, UK

Karen Lu MD Professor of Gynecologic Oncology, The University of Texas M.D. Anderson Cancer Center, Houston, Texas, USA

Anneke Lucassen DPhil FRCP Professor in Clinical Genetics, Wessex Clinical Genetics Service, Princess Anne Hospital, Southampton, UK

Karim Meeran MD FRCP Professor of Endocrinology, Charing Cross and Hammersmith Hospitals, London, UK, and Imperial College, London, UK

Fausto Palazzo MS FRCS Consultant Endocrine Surgeon, Hammersmith Hospital, London, UK, and Honorary Senior Lecturer, Imperial College, London, UK

Susan Parry FRACP Gastroenterologist, New Zealand Familial Gastrointestinal Cancer Registry, Auckland City Hospital and Department of Gastroenterology, Middlemore Hospital, Auckland, New Zealand

Kathleen Schmeler MD Assistant Professor of Gynecologic Oncology, The University of Texas M.D. Anderson Cancer Center, Houston, Texas, USA

Huw Thomas MA PhD FRCP Professor of Gastrointestinal Genetics and Consultant Gastroenterologist, Imperial College, St Mark's Hospital, Harrow, UK

Meena Upadhyaya PhD FRCPath Professor of Medical Genetics and Consultant Molecular Geneticist, Institute of Medical Genetics, Cardiff University, Cardiff, UK

Thomas K Weber MD FACS Professor of Surgery and Molecular Genetics, Albert Einstein College of Medicine, New York, USA; Chief of Surgery, Einstein Weiler Hospital, New York, USA

Olivia Will MB ChB MRCS(Eng) Surgical Research Fellow, The Polyposis Registry, St Mark's Hospital, Harrow, UK

John Windsor FRACS MD Professor of Surgery, Department of Surgery, University of Auckland, Auckland, New Zealand

Foreword

Intensive research over the last fifteen years has yielded a vast expansion in our understanding of the role of inheritance and genetics in many cancers. Several inherited conditions have been identified which result in a high risk of various cancers; some of these were previously recognised, but the genetic basis underlying them has now been elucidated.

This knowledge is now entering the sphere of routine clinical care. This raises challenges for clinicians untrained in genetics and unfamiliar with the evolving legal and ethical issues, molecular technology and implications for disease management.

The authors are active researchers and clinicians, and many are non-geneticists who have developed expertise in inherited cancer syndromes occurring in their specialty. As well as outlining fundamental genetic principles, and describing the more common inherited cancer syndromes and their management, they have been asked to look to the future of this exciting and rapidly developing field.

Sue Clark MD FRCS (Gen Surg)
Consultant Colorectal Surgeon and Assistant Director
The Polyposis Registry, St Mark's Hospital, Harrow, UK

Chapter 1

Genetics is not complicated

John Burn MD FRCP FRCPCH FRCOG FMedSci
Professor of Clinical Genetics, Newcastle University
Newcastle upon Tyne, UK

Background

There is something wonderfully simple about writing instructions in a universal alphabet of only four letters that provide descriptive words, all three letters long, for the amino acids which make up the proteins of the body or for the punctuation marks (Table 1). The challenge for the clinician

Table 1. Genetic code - some examples.

Amino acid	DNA base coding sequence
Alanine	GCT, GTT, GTA, GCG
Methionine	ATG
Isoleucine	ATT, ATC, ATA
Lysine	AAA, AAG
Stop codon	TAG, TGA, TAA

is connecting the basic anatomy of genes through to the patient who just told you that they are the third person in the family to have a particular illness, or worse still that they are worried about their risk of a syndrome you have never heard of. Added to this longstanding cause of anxiety is the realisation that there may now be a genetic test for this condition but you are not sure how to organise it.

Clinicians approach problems on a 'need to know' basis and remember information best when it relates to a clinical problem. These introductory pages are a reminder of the basic language needed to make sense of the later sections and are not intended to be comprehensive. A reading list of good genetics textbooks and useful reference sources is provided at the end of the chapter.

Genetic disorders are not rare

There is no doubt that there are many vanishingly rare disorders with a genetic basis, upwards of 6,000 of them. My favourite at the moment is a dominant trait called Birt Hogg Dube syndrome which carries a risk of renal cancer. The fact that there are so many rare disorders contributes to the assertion that this is not a rare problem. A survey in a Canadian population added together all the people who presented with a single gene defect or a major malformation and discovered that one in 20 people will have developed or died from a genetic disorder by the age of 25 years. Add to this the later onset conditions like hereditary breast and colon cancer and the fact that a major disease in a younger person will have a big impact on their whole family and associated clinicians, and it is obvious that, collectively, genetic disorders are very common, especially in developed countries where infectious diseases and malnutrition present fewer problems.

Chromosomes

Long before the recognition of the importance of DNA, early microscopists recognised that the thread-like 'coloured bodies' or chromosomes visible in the nuclei of dividing cells (Figure 1) clearly had

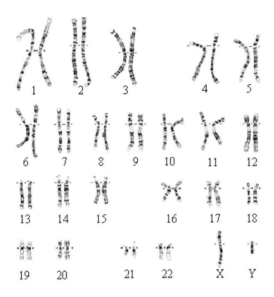

Figure 1. Normal male human karyotype.

something to do with transmission of hereditary information. Surprisingly, it was not until 1956 that it was established that human cells contain 46 chromosomes, by which time the anatomy had become clearer.

Structure

Each of the 23 pairs of chromosomes is a long DNA molecule, coiled around histone proteins, then coiled and coiled again (Figure 2). When we see the familiar karyotype (Figure 1) in textbooks we are looking at a brief moment when the chromosomes have become supercoiled and are in a duplicated state. The cells are poisoned with colchicine to hold them at this point, when they are most easily examined and identified, based on the characteristic banding pattern produced by the physical and chemical interaction of the chromosomes with Giemsa stain.

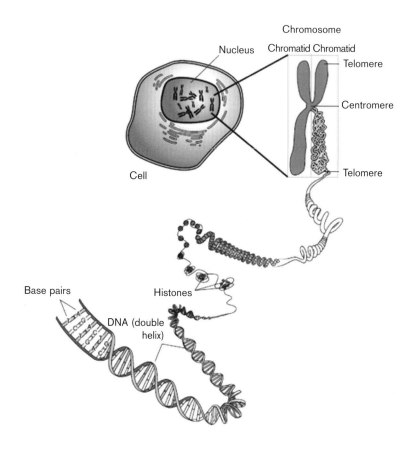

Figure 2. Chromosome structure. *Reproduced under the GNU Free Documentation License (GFDL). (http://creationwiki.org/GNU_Free_Documentation_License).*

It is this banding which gives rise to the positional nomenclature of genes within chromosomes. For example the *APC* gene is positioned at 5q21. This means that it is on chromosome 5, on the long arm of the chromosome (q denotes locations on the long arm of a chromosome, and p locations on the short arm). 21 denotes band 1 in region 2, these locations being defined by the visible banding of the chromosome. This is shown in Figure 3.

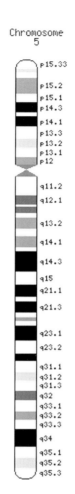

Figure 3. Ideogram of chromosome 5.

In years to come, the 'old fashioned' photograph of matching pairs of chromosomes will give way to a synthetic picture constructed by breaking up a person's DNA and hybridising it to short fragments of the genome arranged on a slide. By competing the patient's DNA with a population sample it becomes possible to identify missing bits and extra bits. This technique is rapidly falling in price and is extremely sensitive - in some cases too sensitive. It turns out that humans have chunks of DNA which can be repeated multiple times without clinical effect, so in future there will be much debate about 'chromosomal variants of uncertain significance'.

Conversely, tiny deletions and duplications which are significant will potentially lead us to genes of clinical importance in certain clinical situations. The most dramatic example in colorectal surgical history was the case report of a man with a chromosome 5 deletion and learning disability who also suffered from familial adenomatous polyposis (FAP), an observation which led to the identification of the location of the causative gene and shortly thereafter the *APC* gene itself.

Genes

Often a gene and the protein that it codes for will have the same name. In order to differentiate them italics are used when referring to the gene, and not when referring to the resulting protein (e.g. the *APC* gene codes for the APC protein).

We use the word 'gene' in two interchangeable ways. It can refer to a section of one of the 23 pairs of chromosomes or it can refer to a faulty segment of DNA which results in a disease. Thus, we speak of the *K-ras* gene, or more precisely the *K-ras* gene locus and we speak about the 'gene' responsible for FAP, which refers to a defective copy or allele of the *APC* gene on chromosome 5. When we use the terms dominant and recessive we are discussing alleles at a particular locus.

Dominant or recessive?

When Mendel solved the puzzle of inheritance with his pea plants, he coined the terms dominant and recessive to describe the two basic types of genes, or 'factors' as he called them. As the name suggests, a dominant gene manifests itself in the presence of a recessive gene. The effect of recessive genes, on the other hand, are only seen when there are two copies present.

The situation is further confused by the use of the term dominant to refer to a clinical phenotype or syndrome. Until his death in 2008, Victor McKusick spent over 40 years compiling his textbook, *Mendelian Inheritance in Man*, which has become a free online resource (www.ncbi.nlm.nih.gov/sites/entrez?db=omim). The many thousands of dominant and recessive phenotypes are catalogued along with links to causative genes where known. Many of these phenotypes earn their title on the basis of inheritance pattern. Classically, a dominant trait will be transmitted to half, on average, of the offspring of an affected individual. If a characteristic pattern runs through three generations, this is taken as strong evidence of a dominant gene defect. Recessive gene defects are characterised by occurring in one generation, affecting on average one in four of siblings. This is because each parent is a carrier and each has a half chance of passing on the defective gene so a child has half of a half, or a quarter chance, of receiving two defective copies and developing the disease.

In the field of colon cancer FAP is a classic dominant and mutY human homologue (*MYH*)-associated polyposis or MAP is a classic recessive. It is of historical interest that the term 'familial' used to be synonymous with what we now call recessive traits while 'hereditary' refers to dominant traits. The surgeons responsible for coining the term FAP were clearly unaware of this usage; it should have been HAP!

When family trees are examined in close-up many exceptions emerge. The most obvious in these days of reduced family size and rare cousin marriage is that most examples of recessive and dominant inheritance will be isolated cases. Many dominant traits which are not compatible with reproduction are never seen in two generations.

New mutations

Some, or in some conditions all, cases occur as new mutations. When this is diagnosed it used to be commonplace to reassure parents that this would not happen again. In about 1% of cases this proved to be incorrect because the mutation giving rise to the disease had occurred in an ovary or testis with the result that the parent could produce multiple gametes carrying the same mutation.

Consanguinity

The converse situation can occur in inbred families or where there is a relatively common recessive gene in a population. Under these circumstances an affected person with the recessive disease might meet a carrier of that same gene defect. The affected person must pass on the defective recessive gene and there is a half chance of their partner doing the same with the result that half of their children develop the disease and the recessive trait appears to be behaving as a dominant trait.

Founder mutations

Some mutations are particularly common in distinct populations, and can be traced back to an individual from whom the population has arisen. This phenomenon is particularly manifest in isolated communities.

Interpretation

With the emergence of molecular genetic analysis, most of these errors of interpretation are being corrected but new complexity emerges. It is possible for some mutations in a gene to act in a dominant fashion, whereas others are only pathological in the presence of a second defective allele and are, therefore, classified as recessive. Many phenotypes turn out to be the result of defects in a host of different genes. Sometimes these turn out to be part of a pathway or involve proteins which work together. The mismatch repair proteins are an excellent example of a group of genes whose products are assembled into a complex piece of molecular machinery involved in DNA repair. Mutation in any of the key genes can disrupt this process.

The language of molecular diagnostics

Having established clinically that a patient has sufficient grounds for requesting gene sequencing, the growing challenge is interpretation of the results. As with any emerging field, an extensive and evolving terminology has developed. In many cases, an expert interpretation is required but this will decline as the concepts become absorbed into routine practice.

There are around 24,000 genes scattered across the human chromosomes and diagnostics is focused on around three or four hundred of these though the number is growing steadily.

Exons, introns and splicing

Sequence alterations occur in coding regions of the cell's DNA known as exons. Alterations in non-coding regions, referred to as introns, are traditionally interpreted to be of no functional significance. However, in recent years intron sequence alterations have come under increasing scrutiny for their possible association with human disease including cancer.

The parts of the genes which attract major interest are the exons, the coding segments which are assembled to produce the full message. As a gene is transcribed into RNA, a splicing mechanism recognises the junctions between exons and introns and cuts out the intronic segments allowing the RNA to be assembled. There is a major physiological process called alternative splicing which results in many, sometimes hundreds, of different versions of a gene product depending on which exons are included in the message.

If there is a mutation in the splice recognition sites, which may be in the exon itself or in the neighbouring intron, defective splicing occurs which may mean a section of the gene is left out or that some or all of an intron is included, both of which are usually disruptive.

Mutations

There are five major types of spelling mistake in the exons (Table 2 and Figure 4).

Table 2. Types of mutation.

Mutation	DNA base change	Amino acid change
Conservative	ATT → ATA	Isoleucine - no change
Missense	ATT → ATG	Isoleucine → methionone
Nonsense	AAA → TAA	Lysine → 'stop'

Conservative base changes

These have no effect on the amino acid sequence of the protein product. This is because the 20 amino acids are represented by sets of three letters in the DNA. As the alphabet has four letters, A, C, G and T there are 64 different combinations. This is called the degenerate code because in some cases the last letter of the three makes no difference to the amino acid incorporated into the polypeptide chain. Thus, a change in that third base makes no difference and is clinically neutral, unless it separately affects the splice mechanism.

Missense mutations

These usually involve changing a single base with the result that a different amino acid is put into the final protein. Many missense mutations are irrelevant and represent a major burden on the genetics services who must try to decide whether such a change (a 'variant of unknown significance') has any clinical significance. Some of these will turn out to have a minor effect and influence the course of the disease but are not the primary cause. Others cause massive disruption to function.

The classic example is the single base change in the beta globin gene, which replaces glutamic acid with valine at position six. The result is that the finished haemoglobin molecules are highly likely to stick together when the oxygen tension falls and the classic 'sickle cell' distortion of the red cells leads to the vascular compromises and anaemia of sickle cell disease. Carriers of this change are resistant to cerebral malaria and so have become very numerous in malaria zones, reaching one in three people in the Rift Valley of Africa, despite the severe morbidity and mortality in children who are homozygous for the mutation. It has been estimated that there are 15,000 missense mutations to be discovered in the BRCA1 and BRCA2 genes, most of which will be of no great clinical significance. Attempts are underway to develop a Human Variome Project, which will allow international pooling of data to help solve this problem.

Nonsense mutations

These mutations convert an amino acid into a 'full stop' resulting in premature termination of the polypeptide chain and usually major disruption of function. They are sometimes referred to as truncating mutations.

Deletions

Loss of DNA might affect whole chromosomes or might involve three bases resulting in loss of a single amino acid. The common cystic fibrosis gene defect carried by almost one in 30 British people involves loss of the 508th amino acid from the chloride channel gene *CFTR*.

Frameshift mutations

Loss or gain of any number of bases not divisible by three results in alteration of the reading frame. This is illustrated in Figure 4. In some cases a stop codon is altered, so the polypeptide chain gets longer. More often, there is a premature chain termination. If this occurs before what should have been the last exon, a physiological process called nonsense-mediated decay leads to the RNA being destroyed. This can mitigate the damage caused by the mutation, especially if the polypeptide chain forms part of a polymer where an abnormal gene product is very disruptive.

GTT ATG AAA AAA ATA GCT → alanine-methionine-lysine-lysine isoleucine-alanine

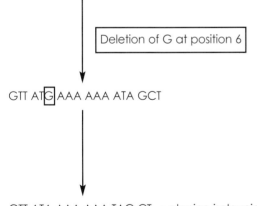

Deletion of G at position 6

GTT ATG AAA AAA ATA GCT

GTT ATA AAA AAA TAG CT → alanine-isoleucine-lysine-lysine-STOP

Figure 4. Frameshift mutation.

We are working on routine techniques that can detect nonsense-mediated decay by analysis of the RNA product of important genes. The idea is that demonstration of loss of one allele is a quick way of determining that there is an important mutation somewhere in that person's gene, which can be identified by sequencing.

Describing mutations

There is an evolving and confusing variety of ways of documenting mutations. These can either involve describing the alteration of the DNA bases (e.g. c.1061A>T, meaning that at base 1061 in the coding DNA adenine has been replaced by thymine) or of the resulting amino acid change (e.g. p.gln581X, meaning that the glycine at the 581st amino acid position has been replaced by a stop codon).

Methylation - the fifth base

When embryonic cells undergo differentiation into the different cell types of the body, genes are switched on and off in specific sequence. A key element of this process involves addition of a methyl group to specific cytosines. It is probably best to consider methyl cytosine as the fifth letter in the DNA alphabet. In the field of colorectal cancer, the situation where this has greatest effect is in relation to the promoter of the *MLH1* gene which can be silenced by methylation leading to loss of mismatch repair gene function; around one in six sporadic colorectal cancers have this basis.

Imprinting

A special aspect of this process is described as imprinting. Around a hundred genes, many involved in critical aspects of growth and development, are selectively methylated so that only one copy of the gene is active. Either the maternal or the paternal version of the gene in question is silenced at the time of gamete formation and remains methylated throughout life. Only when that person comes to produce gametes will the imprint be wiped off and a new imprint applied.

Environmental influence

The study of methylation and its effects is a major area of research because it provides a way in which environment and genes can interact.

For example, a major source of methyl groups needed to methylate genes is acquired from maternal dietary folate. Poor maternal nutrition can affect an individual throughout life. In general terms, a fetus is set up for the world they can expect to face, so that a deprived fetus who is then exposed to high calorie intake is particularly vulnerable to hypertension, obesity and diabetes. There is growing evidence that some degree of this imprint persists into subsequent generations, making the 'nature versus nurture' debate rather more complex.

Mosaicism

This phenomenon occurs when a new mutation arises not in a gamete or single cell embryo, but a little later in development. The result is that some parts of the individual's body are formed from cells carrying the mutation (i.e. will have the disease in question) but the rest are not. This can cause considerable clinical and diagnostic confusion.

Individuals have been reported with FAP who have a classical polyposis phenotype, with the causative mutation present in normal bowel mucosa found between polyps, not apparent in the white blood cells usually used for mutation detection. Another confusing scenario occurs when an apparently healthy parent produces a child with an autosomal dominant disorder. The simplest explanation of this is that the child has a new mutation. An alternative is that the parent is a mosaic, with gonads affected, but the tissues where the gene normally causes disease (e.g. colon in FAP) are not affected. It is for this reason that it is important to screen the siblings of probands who appear to carry a new mutation.

The future

In recent years it has become clear that the DNA in the long gaps between genes is of major importance. Many thousands of short RNA molecules are produced which are 'non-coding'. That is to say, they are not translated into proteins but act instead to control the activity and levels of expression of the major structural genes. The true clinical significance of this class of genetic information is just beginning to emerge but will be of great importance in the future.

The last few months have seen the identification of ten genes that contribute to familial risk of colorectal cancer. While around 5% of colorectal cancer is attributable to a single gene defect, twin studies indicate up to 30% of the cause of colorectal cancer is genetic. The challenge will be to identify all of the genes involved in this broader predisposition and develop rapid molecular analysis and algorithms to enable clinicians to offer useful intervention based on these tests. Unfortunately, there will be a rush to exploit these discoveries and provide the 21st century equivalent of the brown bottles sold as a cure for all ills by the forerunners of the pharmaceutical industry.

Key points

♦ While individual inherited cancer syndromes are rare, together they make up a substantial disease burden, which particularly affects younger adults.

♦ The nomenclature used to describe the position of genes on a chromosome is based on the appearance of the chromosome.

♦ While the concept of dominant and recessive inheritance is straightforward, other factors may cause confusion.

♦ Several types of mutation can occur, with different resulting effects and differences in ease of detection.

♦ It is not just DNA sequence that is important - epigenetic phenomena such as imprinting can have profound effects.

Further reading

1. Mueller RF, Young ID. *Emery's Elements of Medical Genetics*. Churchill Livingstone, 2001.
2. Harper PS. *Practical Genetic Counselling*, 6th Ed. London: Arnold Publishers, 2004.
3. Firth HV, Hurst JA. *Oxford Desk Reference Clinical Genetics*. Oxford: Oxford University Press, 2005.
4. Lalloo F, Kerr B, Friedman JM, Evans GR. *Risk Assessment and Management in Cancer Genetics*. Oxford: Oxford University Press, 2005.
5. Read A, Donnai D. *New Clinical Genetics*, 1st Ed. Scion Publishing Ltd, 2007.

Chapter 2

Genetics and cancer

Thomas K Weber MD FACS
Professor of Surgery and Molecular Genetics, Albert Einstein College of
Medicine, New York, USA
Chief of Surgery, Einstein Weiler Hospital, New York, USA

Background

It is generally understood that cancer is a 'genetic disease'. However, in that simple expression, 'a genetic disease', is a world of vitally important information for both patients and clinicians, as well as many unanswered questions. While cancer genetics is a vast and potentially intimidating subject, its basic principles are readily accessible and often clinically relevant. Limits to knowledge about cancer genetics may compromise the quality of care provided by clinicians as well as confuse and frustrate patients. Examples include clinical screening protocols for many solid tumours such as colorectal and breast cancer. Patient selection and optimal utilization of these life-saving protocols are facilitated by a basic knowledge of cancer genetics. Equally important, these same protocols also require the clinician to acquire and use family history information. Obtaining family history of cancer information from patients is an important component of good practice and is a vital tool that is often neglected [1]. Similarly, understanding both the benefits and limitations of genetic testing and the new, state-of-the art targeted molecular therapies for cancer also requires a basic working knowledge of the molecular genetics of cancer.

The goal of this book is to provide busy clinicians with a useful introduction to clinical cancer genetics in the 21st century. In this chapter we will present a review of the basic principles and molecular building blocks of cancer genetics. Subsequent chapters will review a range of specific hereditary cancers in more detail. The purpose of the material in this chapter is to make the more detailed information in the rest of the book more accessible, understandable and clinically useful.

We will first explain a crucial distinction between germline and somatic cancer genetics. We will then look briefly at the primary patterns of inheritance of cancer syndromes. This will be followed by a review of the key concepts surrounding oncogenes, tumour suppressor genes, DNA damage response genes and genomic instability in cancer. The role of non-inherited cancer tissue-specific genetic changes, referred to as somatic genetic alterations, will also be considered. This will allow us to review another important topic, multi-step carcinogenesis. The types of mutations that cause cancer, loss of heterozygosity, genotype and phenotype will be discussed and the distinction between mutations and polymorphisms will be explained.

Not every aspect of cancer predisposition, development and outcome is directly linked to an individual's germline or tumour DNA sequence. Other factors in the cells of our bodies and the wider environment in which we live also affect the expression of genes. We will take a brief look at some of these factors including RNA, epigenetics and stem cells. The importance of family history information and the opportunities presented by the Human Variome Project [2] will also be discussed.

Germline and somatic genetic alterations

It is important to clarify that cancer genetics includes two related but profoundly different genetic concepts: namely, germline genetic changes and somatic genetic changes.

Germline mutation

The term germline mutation refers to alterations in an individual's DNA that was present at embryogenesis and affects all of the person's cells including, importantly, the egg or sperm cells which are referred to as gametes. Because germline genetic changes are present in the gametes they are potentially passed on to (or inherited by) the person's offspring. Much of what we review in this and subsequent chapters will focus on these germline changes and the hereditary cancer syndromes associated with them.

Somatic mutation

The term somatic is derived from the Greek word *somatikos* meaning 'of the body'. In the context of cancer, somatic genetic changes are alterations that occur in the DNA of individual cells of a particular tissue of the body; somatic mutation may result in the development and or progression of a cancer. Examples include genetic alterations in the cells lining the colon, leading to colon cancer; cells lining the ducts of the breast, leading to breast cancer; or the cells lining the bronchus of the lung, resulting in a lung cancer. Another very useful concept is the fact that somatic genetic changes also play a role in the initiation and progression toward cancer of pre-malignant lesions such as colonic adenomatous polyps. We will look at this process, often referred to as multi-step carcinogenesis in more detail below.

Again, in contrast to germline genetic alterations, somatic alterations are not detected in the cells of unaffected tissues of the body or even cells nearby the pre-malignant lesion or eventual cancer. Also importantly, these somatic alterations do not affect the gametes or germ cells. This means that somatic genetic alterations in human cancers are not passed on to offspring. However, potentially confusing is the fact that somatic genetic changes may occur in human cancers in the very same genes that do sometimes also play a role in inherited cancer syndromes. So, for example, somatic genetic changes in the *APC* gene are a very frequent finding in sporadic (non-hereditary) colorectal adenomas and cancers. These somatic *APC* gene alterations are not passed on or inherited. However, a small but important proportion of human colorectal cancers occur in patients with inherited germline *APC* gene mutation, who have familial adenomatous polyposis (FAP) [3].

Inherited cancer syndromes

Many decades before the Human Genome Project, the complete sequencing of the human genome and the launch of the Human Variome Project [2], it was known by clinicians as well as astute family historians that a number of human cancers do occur with greater frequency in some families. Such patterns are described initially as familial cancer and may eventually be described as hereditary if a specific pattern of inheritance can be verified. In some families the pattern of cancer incidence across multiple generations follows the basic principles of inheritance first described by the Austrian monk Gregor Mendel. In the Mendelian genetic model the physical traits or phenotype of an individual are the result of the aggregate influence or expression of approximately 24,000 genes that direct the millions of cells of our body. Each gene or locus has two copies (alleles), one derived from the mother (maternal) and one from the father (paternal). There are two principal forms of Mendelian inheritance: autosomal dominant and autosomal recessive.

Autosomal dominant cancer syndromes

In autosomal dominant cancer syndromes only one altered allele (maternal or paternal) is required to significantly increase the individual's risk of developing the associated cancer phenotype. Because mutation of only one of the two alleles is required to cause such syndromes the altered allele is said to be dominant, hence the term autosomal dominant inheritance. In addition, because only one of the two alleles is required to be altered in autosomal dominant cancer syndromes there is a 50% chance that the offspring of parents, one of whom has the cancer predisposition gene, will inherit that trait (Figure 1a).

If successfully transmitted the child is then referred to as a carrier of the cancer-causing allele. Because only one mutated cancer allele is required to cause the cancer and that mutated allele is different than the normal (or wild-type), the carrier is referred to as heterozygous at the specific gene or genetic locus in question. Importantly, simply carrying an autosomal dominant cancer susceptibility gene does not guarantee that the carrier will develop the cancer associated with that gene. The likelihood of a

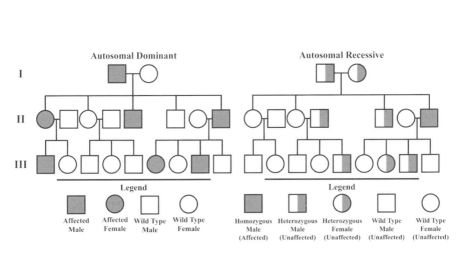

Figure 1. Dominant and recessive pedigrees.

specific mutation resulting in the development of the cancer in question is described by the term penetrance. The penetrance of the cancer-associated mutation will depend on many factors including the normal function of the altered gene and the extent to which the mutation alters the ability of the protein product of the gene to perform its normal function. Provided the mutated gene is highly penetrant, up to 50% of the offspring may demonstrate the cancer phenotype (i.e. 100% of carriers). Examples of autosomal dominant hereditary cancer syndromes include FAP, BRCA1 and 2-associated breast cancer and Lynch syndrome.

Recessively inherited cancer syndromes

Not all hereditary cancer syndromes follow the autosomal dominant pattern of inheritance. Some follow what is referred to as recessive inheritance. In autosomal recessive disorders the disease trait can only be expressed when both the maternal and paternal allele contribution to the child carry the alteration or mutation that predisposes the individual to the disease.

Both alleles must be altered in recessive disorders; if both alleles are the same with respect to the disease causing alteration geneticists refer to this sameness as homozygous at the locus in question. If both alleles are affected, but with a different mutation at each, the term compound heterozygote is used.

The requirement for both alleles to be affected in recessive disorders means of course both parents must carry at least one copy, that is they both must be heterozygous for the trait (i.e. an unaffected carrier) or one or both of them may be affected (homozygous or compound heterozygous). In contrast to the 50% probability of effective transmission of autosomal dominant traits to offspring the probability of transmission in recessive disorders is only 25% if both parents are unaffected carriers (Figure 1b).

Detecting the presence of a recessive disorder can be very challenging especially in societies where small families with two or less children per generation are common. The requirement for both parents to carry the trait means expression of the disease in multiple successive generations is far less likely than in autosomal dominant syndromes. The classic family history pattern of recessive disorders is the observation of a single generation in which multiple individuals are affected. Though relatively rare, examples of autosomal recessive disorders associated with increased cancer incidence include Bloom syndrome, ataxia telangiectasia and MYH-associated polyposis.

In summary, many human malignancies occur in familial patterns that are consistent with the principles of Mendelian inheritance. Specific knowledge of autosomal dominant and recessive hereditary cancer syndromes will help clinicians to identify these families and direct increased cancer surveillance to them. Knowledge of the basic principles of Mendelian genetics will also facilitate the discovery of new familial and hereditary cancer syndromes. Success in these efforts requires diligent attention to patient family history information.

The molecular genetics of cancer

You need not know anything about the existence of DNA or RNA to be able to identify a potential inherited cancer family and make life-saving recommendations regarding their cancer screening and surveillance care. However, dramatic insights into the molecular genetic basis for both inherited cancer syndromes and sporadic cancer initiation and progression have been made over the past two decades. In this section we will review the fascinating story of the discovery and basic principles of oncogenes and tumour suppressor genes.

The oncogene story: a brief version

In 1910, Peyton Rous, working at the Rockefeller Institute in New York demonstrated that soft tissue sarcomas in chickens could be transmitted from one animal to another using extracts from the sarcoma of the first animal injected into the second animal. This basic experiment had been done before. Rous's unique contribution was to demonstrate, using filter papers and microscopy, that the sarcoma extracts he used were cell free [4]. Rous speculated that these results suggested an infectious mechanism for the development of cancer, at least in the animals studied.

There was tremendous resistance to the idea that cancer could be caused by infectious agents. This resistance was fuelled by the fact that Rous's experiments offered no evidence for what the infectious agent might actually be. At the time, knowledge of viruses was largely speculative. However, ultimately the true identity of the infectious agent responsible for the cancer transmission observed by Rous was found to be a virus and ultimately an RNA virus. The RNA viruses are able to reproduce using the nuclear machinery of the host cell. Further extraordinary experimental work demonstrated that a specific segment of the viral RNA genome was responsible for causing the cancers observed in chickens by Rous. Strains of the virus lacking in that specific RNA sequence were unable to cause sarcoma transformation. The specific RNA sequence responsible for the cancer transformation observed by Rous was termed a viral oncogene and named *v-src*; a viral gene responsible for sarcoma.

There is more to this fascinating story. In the mid 1970s, scientists made the profound discovery that the cancer-causing retroviral genes discovered in the Rous sarcoma virus and other avian cancer viruses were remarkably similar to genes that exist in the normal animal genome. In fact, the RNA viral oncogenes were actually slight variations of the same genes identified in normal cells. In the case of the viral *v-src* gene its normal counterpart in animal cells was identified and referred to as *C-SRC*; the cellular counterpart of the sarcoma viral oncogene.

As a group, the cellular counterparts of the viral oncogenes were referred to as proto-oncogenes. Many proto-oncogenes normally code for enzymes and other protein products that regulate cell growth. Proto-oncogenes that are mutated or otherwise altered to facilitate malignant transformation often act by increased stimulation of growth. Oncogenic alterations of proto-oncogenes are often referred to as 'gain of function' mutations. These gain of function changes contribute to excessive cell growth and progression toward the cancer phenotype. Many decades following his initial discovery Peyton Rous was awarded the Nobel Prize in 1966 for his seminal contributions to our understanding of viral oncogenesis and human malignancy.

Tumour suppressor genes

A second important group of genes associated with an inherited predisposition to cancer and understanding the process of malignant transformation are the tumour suppressor genes. The tumour suppressor gene story complements, in many respects, the oncogene story described above. In their normal or wild-type state tumour suppressor genes help to control and limit cell growth. Alterations in the DNA sequence or mutations of tumour suppressor genes result in the gene being unable to code for its normal protein product. In many cases this means the protein is not produced at all. In other examples the protein is produced but compromised in size or otherwise altered so that it cannot perform its normal growth regulating function. In the tumour suppressor gene model the mechanism of initiating cancer is loss of gene function. Loss of tumour suppressor gene function results in loss of cellular growth control, a fundamental characteristic of cancer cells.

Knudson's hypothesis

Our first insights into the tumour suppressor gene model of cancer initiation began with the investigation of retinoblastoma. In the early 1970s, Alfred Knudson focused his attention on this relatively rare but devastating childhood disease characterised by the development of a malignant tumour of the retina. Knudson observed that retinoblastoma occurred with increased frequency in some families but also appeared to occur sporadically in families without a history of the disease. Importantly, Knudson observed that in the familial form the disease often affected both of the children's eyes and multiple retinal tumours were possible in each eye. In contrast, in the sporadic form of the disease only one eye was affected, most often by a single retinoblastoma tumour. Knudson also observed that the familial form of the disease tended to occur at a younger age than the sporadic form.

Based on these observations Knudson offered the hypothesis that the development of retinoblastoma required two genetic alterations or 'hits' [5]. This is now known as the Knudson's 'two-hit' hypothesis. Knudson reasoned that in the familial version of the disease the affected child inherited the predisposition from the germline and was born with the first genetic alteration required to cause the disease. Every cell of the child therefore carried the first 'hit'. However, inheritance of this single hit was not sufficient to cause the disease in Knudson's two-hit model. In the model the second hit or genetic alteration was predicted to be a somatic mutation that occurred in a cell of the child's retina, after birth. In contrast, in the sporadic form of the disease both genetic alterations required for retinoblastoma development are somatic events. Neither is inherited. Consistent with Knudson's hypothesis the sporadic form of the disease affects only one eye, results in a solitary tumour and occurs later in life.

While Knudson's ground-breaking hypothesis explained a general mechanism for the incidence of retinoblastoma it took many years before the actual genetic elements involved were identified. Knudson's hypothesis introduced an opportunity for a novel genetic paradigm in cancer that went beyond the oncogenes model. It took over a decade before scientists in multiple independent laboratories identified the precise DNA sequence of the retinoblastoma gene and its exact location on chromosome 13. Not surprisingly, subsequent investigations showed that the function of the retinoblastoma (Rb) gene protein product was cell cycle regulation, an important dynamic in controlling cell growth. The retinoblastoma story powerfully illustrates the value of diligent clinical observation and collaborative efforts between physicians and scientists in order to translate clinical bedside observations into useful fundamental scientific discoveries. Important additional examples of tumour suppressor genes that contribute to cancer incidence include the *APC*, *BRCA1* and *2* and DNA mismatch repair genes.

A confusing aspect of this topic is the fact that mechanistically recessive tumour suppressor gene-associated inherited cancer syndromes, such as retinoblastoma, are transmitted in an autosomal dominant fashion. This seeming paradox is explained by the hypothesis that the inheritance of the first hit, though insufficient to cause disease on its own, is associated with a rate of somatic mutation at the second allele such that cancer incidence fits the dominant familial pattern.

DNA damage response genes

The term DNA damage response genes refers to a very diverse group of genes that have one common characteristic; they all code for protein products that contribute to the cell's ability to identify and correct damage to its DNA. This DNA damage may occur randomly or as a result of exposure to a mutagenic substance from the environment (carcinogens). Compromise or loss of function of any one of these genes is associated with a diverse range of syndromes all of which are in turn associated with increased cancer incidence. These include xeroderma pigmentosum, Fanconi anaemia, Bloom syndrome and ataxia telangiectasia (Table 1).

An extremely important additional group of genes of the DNA damage response type are the DNA mismatch repair genes. Germline mutations in these genes are strongly associated with an increased incidence of hereditary early age onset colorectal and other cancers and are described in more detail in Chapter 6, which focuses on Lynch syndrome.

Table 1. DNA damage response gene syndromes and associated cancers.

Affected gene	Hereditary syndrome	Associated cancer
ATM	Ataxia-telangiectasia	Lymphoma, leukaemia, breast
MRE11A	AT-like disorder	Lymphoma
NBS1	Nijmegen breakage syndrome	Lymphoma
BRCA1	Familial breast cancer 1	Breast, ovarian, prostate, colon
BRCA2	Familial breast cancer 2	Breast (female/male), ovarian, prostate, pancreas
CHK1	None reported	Colorectal and endometrial cancer
CHK2	Li-Fraumeni syndrome	Breast, lung, colon, urinary bladder, testis
p53	Li-Fraumeni syndrome	Sarcoma, breast, brain, leukaemia
RECQL2	Werner syndrome	Various cancers
RECQL3	Bloom syndrome	Leukaemia, lymphoma
RECQL4	Rothmund-Thomson syndrome	Osteosarcoma
DNA MMR • MSH2 • MLH1 • PMS2 • MSH6	Lynch syndrome	Colon, rectum, endometrium, ovarian, urinary organs, gastric, skin
p16	Familial melanoma	Melanoma, pancreas
RB	Familial retinoblastoma	Retinoblastoma, osteosarcoma
CSA, CSB	Cocayne's syndrome	Skin
XPA-XPG	Xeroderma pigmentosum	Skin

Genomic instability

Genomic instability refers to a number of different phenomena that characterise variations from normal in chromosome number, structure and DNA sequence fidelity in cancer cells. These abnormal characteristics result from failures in the cancer cell's ability to maintain DNA sequence fidelity and or accurately replicate and pair chromosomes during mitotic cell division. For our purposes we will briefly consider three components of genomic instability in human cancer: aneuploidy, chromosomal instability and microsatellite instability.

Aneuploidy and chromosome instability

Aneuploidy refers to the consistent observation in the majority of human solid tumours that the number of chromosomes observed in the cancer cell nucleus is different than the normal diploid complement of 46. Aneuploid cancer cells have been observed to have as many as 70, 80 or even more chromosomes within the nucleus. This consistent variation in chromosomal number variation from normal is referred to as chromosomal instability or CIN. Looking more closely, CIN has been shown to be characterised by multiple specific structural abnormalities of the chromosomes in cancer cells. These include translocations where whole segments of a chromosome move to a different abnormal location on the same chromosome or another chromosome, inversions where the chromosomal segment is flipped and inserted 'backwards' into the chromosome, duplications of large segments or entire chromosomes and finally, deletions resulting in the loss of microscopically visible segments of a chromosome representing the loss of DNA containing many genes.

Loss of heterozygosity

Loss of heterozygosity (LOH) is an important concept based on the observation that often, each parental allele (maternal and paternal) at any given genetic locus differs slightly from the other. Because of these slight differences in DNA sequence between the two alleles the situation is often described as heterozygous at that locus. Should a pathologic DNA sequence alteration take place for whatever reason at either one of these wild-type alleles the situation for that gene remains heterozygous. However, for the tumour suppressor gene model described above, that pathologic alteration will not, on its own, cause the associated disease or cancer. This is because the tumour suppressor gene model is mechanistically recessive. The remaining wild-type allele must also be altered or lost for the full loss of gene function required to allow malignant transformation to occur. When the loss of this remaining wild-type allele occurs leaving only the disease-associated mutated allele this is referred to as reduction to homozygosity.

When a cell loses a chromosome or part thereof, it might expose the fact that the other copy of the gene is defective or missing. For example, if a person inherits a faulty version of the *APC* gene, their cells are all prone to abnormal cell division but this is suppressed by the remaining copy of the gene. Only when that remaining copy is lost by a cell will tumour development proceed. This often occurs as a result of loss of a section of chromosome during cell division.

This tendency, for chromosome loss to lead to the appearance of cancer, is exploited in 'gene hunting'. When a chromosome, or part of it, is lost by a cell, one copy of all the DNA around the 'disease gene' is also lost. There are now hundreds of thousands of recognised variants along the length of all our chromosomes, usually in the form of a harmless single letter change or single nucleotide polymorphism (SNP) so all people will have differing letter sequences on their chromosome pairs. The technical term is to be heterozygous for a particular marker or SNP. If a person has a single letter defect in their *APC* gene, then loses the other chromosome 5, they will lose one copy of all the SNPs in the vicinity of the gene. This loss of heterozygosity thus becomes a tell-tale sign of the likely location of the gene with the inherited defect. Clearly there could be coincidental loss of a variety of chromosomes but by pooling many tumours the areas with consistent loss of heterozygosity become a reliable indicator of a disease gene.

Microsatellite instability

Microsatellite instability refers to characteristic alterations in short repetitive sequences of DNA known as microsatellites. Microsatellite instability is frequently referred to in the literature as MSI. In the cancer context MSI was first described in DNA isolated from colorectal cancers resected from patients who were members of the hereditary colorectal cancer syndrome known as Lynch syndrome or hereditary non-polyposis colorectal cancer (HNPCC). As MSI takes place in tumour DNA these DNA changes are somatic in nature. The discovery of MSI was crucial and contributed directly to the eventual discovery of the role of germline alterations in the DNA mismatch repair genes in Lynch syndrome. MSI is not just an esoteric detail in the genetics of cancer. Positive MSI status in human colorectal cancer has been associated with characteristic changes in tumour pathology, natural history and response to therapy.

Mutations and polymorphisms

Oncogenes and tumour suppressor genes cause or contribute to cancer initiation when the expression of their normal protein products is altered in a way that affects or eliminates their function. Using the term pathogenic mutation to describe a DNA sequence alteration implies the alteration is pathologically significant, meaning the alteration is directly linked to disease. Not all DNA sequence alterations are necessarily linked to cancer or disease causation. Importantly, discussions of mutations may pertain to heritable germline mutations or somatic mutations that only take place in the cells of the tumour. Polymorphisms are DNA sequence alterations that are judged by studied consensus to be of no functional significance and are therefore interpreted as non-disease-causing or non-pathogenic.

Multi-step carcinogenesis

We have described the role of oncogenes and tumour suppressor genes, as well as the specific group of DNA damage control genes and genomic instability in the context of inherited cancer syndromes. Interestingly, the majority of breast, colon and all other solid tumour malignancies do not occur in familial patterns and are not the result of known, identifiable inherited mutations. However, many solid tumour cancers including colon cancer in particular, are characterised by multiple somatic genetic alterations. As noted above somatic genetic alterations occur only in the tumour cells and are not passed on through the germline or inherited. These multiple steps to cancer initiation and progression are referred to as multi-step carcinogenesis.

The adenoma to carcinoma sequence in colorectal cancer

There is ample evidence that multi-step carcinogenesis occurs in numerous human cancers; however, the most extensive documentation of this phenomenon has been demonstrated in colorectal cancer.

Current thinking accepts that the overwhelming majority of colorectal cancers begin as small benign polyps. Histologically these abnormal growths are described as adenomatous. In their earliest form they can be observed microscopically and are referred to as aberrant crypt foci. These often continue to grow into readily visible polyps. The observation, collection and molecular analysis of these polyps is greatly facilitated by screening and diagnostic endoscopy (colonoscopy). Importantly, there is no parallel tissue sampling procedure for other solid tumours such as breast, prostate or lung cancer. The molecular analysis of colorectal cancer was pioneered by Vogelstein and associates [6]. The contributions of these investigators to our understanding of colorectal cancer multi-step carcinogenesis are so pivotal that graphic depictions of the cellular process are often referred to as 'Vogelgrams'.

An initial observation by Vogelstein was that alterations in the *APC* gene could be demonstrated in 25-30% of adenomas that were still histologically benign. Importantly, the frequency of *APC* alterations was not found to be any higher in invasive colorectal cancers. However distinct, separate LOH alterations were observed on chromosome 17p, and 18q at a high frequency only in invasive cancers, not in the benign polyp precursors. This suggested the observed *APC* alterations in premalignant polyps were an early step and the 17p and 18q alterations were later events associated with polyp growth.

Similarly, alterations in the *RAS* family of oncogenes are relatively rare in small polyps under 1cm in size. In contrast *RAS* alterations are significantly more frequent in larger adenomas suggesting they also contribute to the adenoma growth process and cancer initiation (Figure 2). These findings are consistent with the hypothesis that a series of genetic changes occurs in the affected cells as the polyp grows and progresses from pre-malignant precursor to an invasive malignancy and, in some cases, beyond to distant metastatic lesions that occur elsewhere in the

A guide to cancer genetics in clinical practice

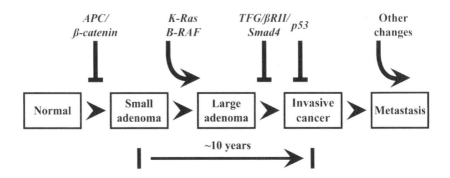

Figure 2. Multiple genetic changes contribute to the adenoma-to-invasive carcinoma sequence in colorectal cancer.

body. Although the colorectal cancer model dominates the multi-step carcinogenesis paradigm, other examples including bladder cancer and skin malignancies have been described.

The insight provided by diligent study of multi-step carcinogenesis has generated many important scientific and clinical advances. Detailed study of the proteins produced by the genes affected in multi-step carcinogenesis provides both diagnostic and therapeutic opportunities. Importantly the somatically mutated cells shed from the mucosal lining of the colon into the faecal stream can be collected and analysed for the precise genetic alterations associated with polyp and or cancer formation. This evolving science has already been integrated into novel polyp and colon cancer detection technologies. These molecular genetic-based approaches hold significant advantages for patients, as these screening modalities, based on faecal samples, are non-invasive. Further detailed study of each gene product involved in the cancer process also provides opportunities to develop targeted molecular therapies. These therapies, based directly on the somatic genetic alterations described by multi-step carcinogenesis, are designed to address the molecular pathway deficiencies or excesses that result from those same somatic mutations.

Epigenetics

The expression of genes and the impact of RNA transcription and translation on the cancer phenotype are also influenced by other factors. Epigenetics refers to all modifications to genes that affect gene expression other than changes in the DNA sequence itself [7]. Epigenetic studies include investigation of the addition of molecules such as methyl groups to the DNA molecule that directly affect gene expression and have been shown to play a role in turning genes 'on' and 'off'. In cancer genetics, some tumour suppressor genes are actually turned off by epigenetic alterations of the gene resulting in loss of the tumour suppressor gene's growth-limiting protein product. Similarly, epigenetic modifications of growth-promoting oncogenes can result in increased production of the growth-promoting protein product of the gene, which can contribute directly to cancer incidence.

The importance of family history and genetic counselling

It is really only in the past 10 to 15 years that contributions by pioneering clinical cancer geneticists such as Henry Lynch (see Chapter 6, Lynch syndrome), Mary Clair King, and Mark Skolnick (see Chapter 7, Breast Cancer), have provided convincing evidence that a percentage of certain cancers such as colorectal and breast cancer, do in fact occur in definable inherited patterns. During this time knowledge of the science of the genetic basis for inherited cancer has also advanced significantly including the discovery of specific inherited germline DNA mutations associated with an increased risk of developing the cancer in question.

As will be seen in successive chapters of this book, basic knowledge of the already described cancer predisposition syndromes is invaluable information for clinicians and patients. This knowledge assists providers in recognising individuals and families that are at significantly increased risk of developing the cancer or cancers associated with the predisposition syndrome. This in turn guides decisions about the optimal timing and methods used to provide appropriate cancer surveillance in these families. In fact, many national and international cancer screening and surveillance guidelines take into account the presence or absence of such cancer family syndromes in their recommendations. Additional potential benefits of identifying cancer-causing germline mutations include directed clinical surveillance for prevention or earliest stage diagnosis, as well as modified or novel molecular-based therapies.

Of course, clinicians and patients cannot benefit from the increased protection afforded by these modified guidelines and recommendations unless there is an awareness of the individual's family history. Busy physicians may be apprehensive about taking the time to secure a family history. However, it is important to note here that a single simple question such as 'Is there any history of cancer in your family?' can open the door to increased awareness of cancer risk and be literally life-saving. Recognition of early age of diagnosis of adult malignancies also suggests the possibility of genetic predisposition and deserves careful follow-up. Equally important, genetic counselling services should be sought whenever personal or family medical history information suggests the presence of a cancer predisposition syndrome [8]. A further important benefit of diligent attention to family history is the opportunity to expand our understanding of relationships between genotype and phenotype and the discovery of new cancer predisposition syndromes and novel genetic elements associated with cancer predisposition.

The future

RNA

As most readers will know there is an important additional component to the DNA to protein product story, namely ribonucleic acid (RNA). RNA plays a crucial role in the genotype to phenotype story by communicating the genetic information of DNA, using messenger RNA (mRNA) molecules to transcribe the DNA message. The mRNA is then used by cellular ribosomes to translate the genetic message into amino acids that are used to build the final protein product coded by the gene. Clearly, opportunities for variation, error and dysfunction exist in the transcription and translation processes. As we move into the 21st century scientific attention is increasingly focused on the regulation of mRNA transcription. This includes the study of special regulatory RNA molecules known as microRNAs [9]. Differential expression and function of microRNA has been observed in association with several human malignancies, and microRNAs are therefore the subject of exciting new efforts to improve our understanding of malignant transformation and design novel effective cancer therapies.

Cancer stem cells

Cancer stem cells are cells found within solid tumours that possess the ability to give rise to all of the different cell types found in the tumour it is derived from. Cancer stem cells differ from other cancer cells in that they are able to generate tumours through processes of self-renewal and differentiation into multiple cell types. This is a vast, exciting and controversial topic that is perhaps outside the bounds of this book. However, the existence of cancer stem cells capable of unique growth and reproductive capabilities compared to their other tumour cell neighbours challenges earlier paradigms of tumour growth described in terms of clonal expansion directed by Darwinian selection. Suffice to say ever increasing evidence of the existence of cancer stem cells suggests we are in the midst of a paradigm shift in how we think about cancer and how we should approach the subject of cancer and genetics [10].

Genotype, phenotype and the Human Variome Project

Genotype refers to the exact DNA sequence of the gene associated with the cancer or other associated disease in question. Phenotype refers to the detailed characteristics of the expression of the disease and in some cases the association of other cancers or diseases with the primary disease and gene under study. Knowledge of the cancer and disease phenotype associated with specific genetic alterations improves our understanding of the relationships between DNA mutations and disease. Progress in this arena also requires diligent documentation of all of the disease manifestations associated with specific mutations. Clearly this is a task that would benefit from standardised systematic approaches, electronic relational databases and a co-ordinated international effort.

The Human Variome Project (HVP) [2] is an international scientific consortium launched in 2007. The HVP's mission is to collect and curate all human genetic variation affecting human health. The goal is to improve health outcomes by facilitating the unification of data on human genetic variation and its impact on human health. Cancer genetics is a major focus of the HVP. A visit to their web site is not only highly informative, it also serves to underscore the clinical and scientific relevance of the subject of this book.

Key points

◆ The distinction between somatic DNA changes in human cancers and heritable germline DNA alterations is important for understanding clinical cancer genetics.

◆ Documentation of family history of cancer is important and can be life-saving.

◆ Autosomal dominant and recessive patterns of inheritance both play a role in inherited cancer.

◆ Genomic instability including chromosomal abnormalities, loss of heterozygosity and microsatellite instability all contribute to cancer initiation and progression.

◆ Multi-step carcinogenesis explains the molecular genetic steps that take place in the development of many cancers including colorectal cancer.

◆ Epigenetics reminds us that many factors, including our environment, can influence gene expression apart from DNA mutations.

◆ The Human Variome Project (www.humanvariomeproject.org) represents an important global effort to understand the full impact of genetic variation on human disease including cancer.

References

1. U.S. Surgeon General Family History Project. http://www.hhs.gov/familyhistory/.

2. The Human Variome Project. *www.humanvariomeproject.org*.

3. Kinzler KW, Vogelstein B. Lessons from hereditary colorectal cancer. *Cell* 1996; 87: 159-70.

4. Rous P. A sarcoma of the fowl transmissible by an agent separable from the tumor cells. *J Exp Med* 1911; 13: 397-411.

5. Knudson AG Jr, Hethcote HW, Brown BW. Mutation and childhood cancer: a probabilistic model for the incidence of retinoblastoma. *Proc Natl Acad Sci* 1975; 72(12): 5116-20.

6. Cahill DP, Kinzler KW, Vogelstein B. Genetic instability and Darwinian selection in tumours. *Trends Cell Biol* 1999; 9: M57-60.

7. Nystrom M, Mutanen M. Diet and epigenetics in colon cancer. *World J Gastroenterology* 2009; 15(3): 257-63.

8. Prucka SK, McIlvried DE, Korf BR. Cancer risk assessment and the genetic counseling process: using hereditary breast and ovarian cancer as an example. *Med Princ Pract* 2008; 17(3): 173-89.

9. Slack FJ, Weidhaas JB. MicroRNA in cancer prognosis. *N Engl J Med* 2008; 359(25): 2720-2.

10. Boman BM, Huang E. Human colon cancer stem cells: a new paradigm in gastrointestinal oncology. *J Clin Oncol* 2009; 26(17): 2828-38.

Chapter 3

Ethical and legal aspects of cancer genetics

Anneke Lucassen DPhil FRCP
Professor in Clinical Genetics
Wessex Clinical Genetics Service, Princess Anne Hospital, Southampton, UK

Background

Developments in genetics have been enormous over the last few decades, and continue to progress at a very rapid pace. The attendant media coverage of the Human Genome Project, discovery of particular disease genes, gene therapy, gene cloning, police databases and so on, has led to a high level of public interest in genetics but also a degree of suspicion of the field as well as variable expectations of what it can actually deliver. This chapter focuses on some of the ethical and legal issues that are encountered in current cancer genetic practice. None of these issues is unique to cancer genetics, or indeed genetics as a whole, but this chapter will highlight some of the ways in which the practice of cancer genetics may raise ethical and legal issues for today's health care professional.

Different members of the same family may have different views about, for example, whether or not to have a genetic test, with its possible attendant feelings of stigmatisation and guilt, to predict their risk of a particular disease. Some may wish to know what their risk of a familial condition is, whereas others positively reject such predictions. The results of a genetic test in one person may apply to other members of that family or be relevant to future generations. Previous generations can also be involved; genetic testing can be done on very small samples which are stable for many years and which may have been originally taken and stored with no intention of a particular test, or stored long after a person has died. Although the result of a genetic test is permanent, in the sense that it cannot be altered by, for example, diet or medication, it is very likely to also be associated with varying degrees of uncertainty; it cannot predict when a particular condition will develop, or even if it will. However, much media reporting of genetics implies it to be a highly determinative and definitive investigation. It is important to remember that a genetic test (usually referring to a DNA test) is just one mode of obtaining genetic information. Such information may also, at times, be derived from for example, biochemical results, clinical information and family history.

Table 1 summarises some of the reasons why ethico-legal issues might arise in practice.

Autonomy in genetics

Over the last 30 years medical practice has placed an increasing emphasis on individual patient rights and confidentiality. Respect for patient autonomy plays a central role in both legal and ethical frameworks governing clinical practice and is a key component of many of the professional codes of practice and guidelines governing modern medicine. This, together with a necessity to foster trust between the patient and health professional, underpins the central role that patient confidentiality plays in today's health care relationships.

Whilst this has been a positive move in many ways and has replaced more paternalistic practices, genetic medicine can challenge the apparent supremacy of an individual patient's autonomy. A genetic test on one person can reveal important information about the health, or risk of ill health, of family members, who might (or might not) want to know this, and who might (or might not) benefit from an intervention (for example, surveillance). A tension arises therefore as genetic medicine, which by definition involves families, has to sit within a modern medical framework that lays huge emphasis on individual autonomy.

Table 1. **Aspects of genetic information that may raise ethico-legal issues.**

It is shared within families:

♦ Results in one person may apply to others who have not asked for a test/future generations.

♦ Results may reveal unexpected knowledge about family relationships, for example, misattributed paternity.

It may predict future health:

♦ A result provides a 'permanent' result that cannot be altered by medication/treatment:

- but often with some degree of uncertainty (for example, a *BRCA1* mutation confers a lifetime risk of ovarian cancer of 40%);

- can do so in people currently well and many years before likely onset of symptoms;

- should parents be able to test their children for adult onset diseases?

It may be regarded as sensitive information:

♦ A result may be associated with perceptions of stigma or feelings of guilt.

♦ Possible insurance/employment consequences.

Has issues of scope:

♦ Can be done from cradle to grave, or from 'sperm to worm'.

♦ Large amount of information from very small sample (e.g. sputum, hair root).

♦ DNA databases or biobanks; long-term storage and ability to test a sample collected for 'other' reasons.

Genetic medicine: a family affair

Today's cancer geneticist has some highly accurate and predictive genetic testing to offer but, in isolation, a genetic test is often not as accurate as if it is combined with familial information. For example, if the familial mutation that is causing a high incidence of young onset breast and ovarian cancer is known then an accurate predictive test can be offered to close, at-risk relatives. Without this knowledge, a high risk of cancer might be confirmed, but cannot be excluded. Even though the pick-up rate of pathogenic mutations has improved dramatically in recent years, a negative gene test in an at-risk person does not exclude familial causes that cannot yet be tested for [1]. Genetic testing for at-risk individuals therefore remains a two-step process: first a pathogenic mutation is sought in an affected relative, and secondly, and only if a mutation is found, is a *predictive* test for *this* mutation offered. Knowledge of, and contact with, affected relatives is therefore a prerequisite for this sort of accurate testing.

Even when genetic testing improves such that the predictive powers of a genetic test might no longer require the prior identification of a mutation in a family member (individual genome sequencing is rapidly becoming a more likely financially viable prospect in the near future), the interpretation of genetic testing will still require knowledge of family history and an awareness of interplay between genetic and environmental and developmental factors. Knowledge of one's family history is not always detailed or accurate and so a certain degree of contact with family members is likely to remain necessary to improve the accuracy of a risk assessment. Most cancer genetics departments will try to confirm diagnoses of key cancers in a family history and this requires consent from individuals concerned. A recent study found that one in five risk assessments, and thus screening recommendations, were altered as a result of family history follow-up [2]. For example, Case history 1 (Table 2) illustrates how other family members are required to make an accurate risk prediction in one person.

Taking a family history identifies others at risk

The family tree is an important clinical tool for answering questions about a patient's risk of developing a genetic disorder and appropriate management. A detailed three or more generation pedigree will usually be taken to examine the pattern and types of cancers within a family. Such records contain sensitive information, including family relationships, the health status of family members and dates of birth and death. The names and contact details of family members may also be recorded to facilitate further investigation. Information about family members is usually gathered from individual patients and recorded without relatives' consent or knowledge. Thus a family tree identifies far more individuals than the initial consultand (individual seeking, or referred for, genetic counselling - not to be confused with proband or index case; the family member through whom a family comes to medical attention).

This highlights a difference between a [cancer] genetic medical record and conventional medical records. The latter carry information on one individual, and rarely detailed identifying information on others. Cancer genetic records are family notes and contain information about a varying number of individuals, some of whom may not know that they are thus recorded (see Case history 1; Table 2). The tacit assumption has been that such data are in the public domain because they have been shared within the family and that explicit consent is therefore not required. The advent of data protection and human tissue legislation and the prospect of nationwide electronic records have caused some unease about the legitimacy and limits of such practice.

These anxieties have been addressed by a working party of the British Society of Human Genetics. A detailed document about consent and confidentiality in genetic practice sought advice from legislative experts and opined that family history details should be seen as 'hearsay' information that is already in the public domain and that such details could be recorded and held without the consent of individuals referred to [3]. Under the Data Protection Act (1998) there may well be a reactive duty to let someone who asks know that their name is recorded in a set of notes, but there is probably no proactive duty to do so [4].

Despite this apparent clarity, it is not always obvious how family history information, usually recorded in the form of a pictorial pedigree, has been compiled. Several different family branches may have contributed different pieces of information, some of which may not be general 'hearsay'. For example, one branch may know that an individual was adopted in or out of the family, or that paternity was not as stated [5]. Alternatively, certain individuals may have been contacted to obtain further details of their

Table 2. Identifying others.

Case history 1

Katy's GP sent her for a colonoscopy because her father was diagnosed with terminal colorectal cancer (CRC) at the age of 46. At 26 Katy's colonoscopy was normal, but the surgeon referred her on to genetics for an assessment of her risk and advice on whether or not she should have regular colonic surveillance. Katy was not aware of any further family history of CRC but knew few details about relatives on her father's side.

Figure 1a shows the family history as identified by Katy. Based on this information, Katy would be judged at 'low to moderate' risk of familial bowel cancer and probably not offered regular colonoscopic surveillance.

Six months later she re-attended with her mother; they had found out more about the paternal family. Katy's paternal aunt was said to have had a liver cancer whilst her paternal grandmother had a gynaecological cancer. This granny had two brothers who both had bowel cancer in their late 40s. Consent to access hospital records and cancer registry records was sought (see Table 3). Figure 1b shows the family history after further details sought and confirmations obtained.

Aunt Kathleen had liver secondaries from an ovarian adenocarcinoma and granny Daisy had a uterine cancer. These cancers in combination with a family history of CRC make a diagnosis of Lynch syndrome very likely (see Chapter 6). Microsatellite studies and immunohistochemistry suggested a germline mutation in *MSH2* and a mutation was confirmed in DNA taken from aunt Kathleen.

Based on this information Katy is now thought to be at high risk and two-yearly colonoscopy would be offered. Research studies into surveillance of ovarian and endometrial cancers could also be discussed.

Predictive genetic testing is now available for Katy and for the other close relatives (including her brother, who was described by both Katy and her mother as 'having his head in the sand') identified through detailed family history taking. The names, dates of birth and town of residence for at least two other individuals at 50% risk were identified.

Table 2. Identifying others *continued*.

Learning points:

Katy's initial family history appeared not to confer a large risk to her. It was only after her own 'research' into her family history that more significant details were discovered. This required contact with other family members and access to their records, archival material and a blood sample for DNA testing. Following the identification of a high risk, other relatives could also be offered a predictive genetic test but it is difficult to know how to approach her brother who appears reluctant to be informed.

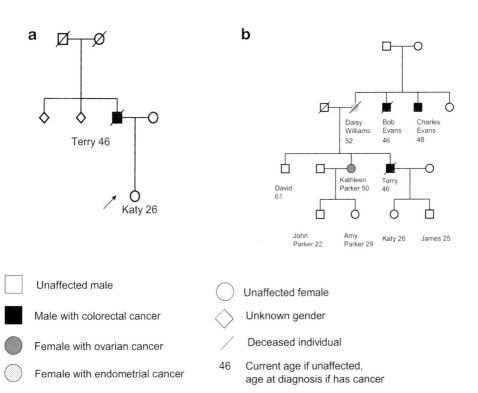

Figure 1. Family history of Case history 1 (Table 2).

cancer diagnoses (see Table 3). Care needs to be taken about if and how such information is recorded and who it is then shared with. It is not unusual for family members or clinicians from other parts of the country to request a copy of a pedigree. Whilst blanket refusal of such requests because of a fear of breaching confidentiality can be unhelpful, sharing should be limited to a 'need to know' basis. These issues will need careful consideration as paper records are converted to electronic records.

Table 3. Consent and medical records of relatives.

- Consent is sought from live relatives by asking consultand to pass request and consent form to relevant people.

- For deceased relatives, there is no statute law governing access to medical records of the deceased (the 1990 Access to Health Records Act governs only legal claims relating to the patient's estate).

- GMC guidelines state that: "After death, doctors still have an obligation to keep personal information confidential". But, they also recommend that "The extent to which confidential information may be disclosed after a patient's death will depend on...the intended use to which the information will be put...and the benefit to the patient's partner or family".

- There is no hierarchy for relatives' consent in access to such information (unlike the hierarchy that the Human Tissue Act 2004 introduced for access to tissue in some circumstances) so a consultand's request should be sufficient. They do not have to be 'next-of kin' (which in any case has no legal definition). There is no requirement for this consent to be in writing [6].

Table 4 summarises some issues to consider when considering at-risk relatives identified through family history taking.

Table 4. Taking a family history of a genetic condition may raise the following issues.

- ◆ Whose responsibility is it to contact relatives known to be at risk?
  - should this be left to the patient?
  - clinicians cannot be expected to trace all relatives in extended families across the world [9] but do they have some moral responsibility to try and contact relatives they know about?
  - does such a duty, if it exists, depend on whether or not there are evidence-based interventions to offer relatives?
- ◆ Do at-risk relatives have a right to know even if the consultand would rather information was not disclosed?
- ◆ Do relatives have a right not to know? If so, how can this best be exercised?
- ◆ Does a genetic test result belong to an individual or to all the family members to whom it might be relevant?

Individual or familial confidentiality?

Despite the modern day importance of confidentiality, it is rarely seen as absolute, and there are both statutory and professional guidelines on exceptions to the duty of confidentiality [7, 8].

Genetic medicine has rarely been mentioned as an exception because few highly predictive genetic tests have been available and there have been relatively few evidence-based interventions. As the evidence basis increases (such as for bowel screening in familial bowel cancer; prophylactic surgery in familial endocrine neoplasia), so does the tension between preserving individual confidentiality and communication of genetic risk to others. Concern for harm to others places a limitation on the duty of confidentiality. Both professional guidelines and UK case law recognise that it can be breached legitimately if considered in the public interest [7, 8]. Recent debate on the disclosure of genetic information to other family members has suggested that it may be appropriate, in rare circumstances, to breach confidentiality if imminent and serious harm can thereby be prevented [9]. The Human Genetics Commission's 2002 report suggested that 'genetic solidarity' and altruism should be promoted [10], and several authors have challenged the supremacy of individual autonomy in genetic medicine and introduced versions of family rather than individual confidentiality [11-13].

For example, the 'joint account model' argues that since genetic information is shared by more than one person, the conventional model of confidentiality should be reversed: the genetic information should be available to all 'account holders' (family members) unless there are good reasons to do otherwise. Thus, genetic information discovered through one person may be considered familial rather than individual and should be shared with others for whom it has relevance, unless there is a very good reason not to [13].

These models are useful in encouraging a different perspective towards genetic information and reflect that most individuals availing themselves of genetic medicine do so with some degree of altruism.

Communication of risk

Once relatives have been identified in a family tree, the clinician may become aware of people who are also at risk of a particular cancer who may not know this themselves. Genetic services in the UK and other countries usually ask an individual to share their genetic information with relatives to whom it may be relevant, and may offer support mechanisms to work with families and their doctors to ensure that people at risk are appropriately informed. Depending on family structure and circumstances such communication can happen effectively, but at other times less so. The latter is difficult to assess because there may be a variety of reasons why relatives do not present to a genetics service. They may have received the relevant information but not wish to pursue genetic testing or they may live in another part of the country or world and therefore their attendance will not come to the attention of the consultand's genetic team.

The non-disclosure of genetic test results has been described and debated, and empirical data have demonstrated a fall off in disclosure with emotional distance [14]. Although a survey of cases in a variety of genetic centres suggested that persistent non-disclosure is rare, this study only examined cases where health care professionals were aware of persistent non-disclosure [15]. The challenge is how to deal with the situation when doctors know the identity of people at risk but consent to communicate that risk has not been obtained. There is no UK case law on this subject, but US courts have made opposing decisions, with one concluding that a doctor should have informed relatives despite the insistence of the affected person that he did not [16, 17]. As noted above, UK professional guidelines tell us that where there is a serious preventable harm confidentiality may be breached, and professionals looking after whole families may feel a moral obligation to inform all the family members who might hold the same genetic information.

Case history 2 (Table 5) describes a case where there was no active refusal, but communication did not occur prior to a (preventable) cancer arising.

The practice of asking patients to communicate their familial risks with their relatives acknowledges the personal and potentially sensitive nature of genetic information and the difficulties of approaching individuals who have not been referred or asked about their own risks. It also arose at a time when there were few interventions or managements to offer those at risk. More recently, as evidence-based interventions for particular genetic conditions have developed, direct communication between the medical professional and family members at risk has been trialled, and found successful and acceptable [18, 19]. However, this has not yet been routinely adopted in UK practice, not least because of the significant workforce and financial implications. Furthermore, these studies relied on the consent of the consultand and do not therefore address the (albeit rare) situation of what to disclose to relatives without such consent. This latter dilemma is more acute when such at-risk relatives are also patients of the same genetics service [20].

Table 5. Non-disclosure.

Case history 2

Denise was referred by the oncologists following the diagnosis of an advanced form of thyroid cancer at the age of 28, because it was thought that others in the family had also had such malignancies. Denise doesn't know that much about her family history as her father died when she was young and her mother lost contact with his family. However, her father, his sister and their father all died in their thirties. These cancers and Denise's age at diagnosis suggest a diagnosis of multiple endocrine neoplasia type 2 (MEN2; see Chapter 9) and gene testing of Denise confirms an inherited mutation in the *RET* proto-oncogene.

Denise has two siblings aged 22 and 25 with whom she is not in regular contact but who live locally and have the same GP. She promises she will get in contact with them and let them know that a highly accurate predictive genetic test is now available to both. Each has a 50% chance of having inherited the gene mutation and a prophylactic thyroidectomy is indicated in gene carriers.

Despite her good intentions, Denise does not get around to doing so. She is ill and wants to concentrate on getting better. Because she has lost contact with her siblings she finds it difficult to know how to approach them.

The genetics department has no addresses for the siblings and asks the help of Denise's GP to locate them. He is, however, reluctant to divulge any information in the absence of Denise's consent. Denise still says that she will do so herself.

A year passes and the geneticist is shocked to hear at a MDT meeting that Denise's brother has now presented aged 23 with advanced metastatic thyroid cancer. He worries that this was preventable and that more should have been done to locate the brother and advise him of his risks.

Table 5. Non-disclosure *continued.*

Learning points:

In this example close relatives were at risk of a serious but preventable condition. Whilst attempts were made to communicate this fact, a more direct approach to Denise's siblings was probably justified. Based on current case law, it is likely that a UK court would determine that the medical professionals could not be legally obligated to contact Denise's relatives, but that they would be allowed to try and contact them. It can certainly be argued that the GP and the genetics service had an ethical obligation to contact Denise's siblings.

Genetic testing of children

Once a disease causing mutation has been identified in a family, it is perhaps not surprising that parents might be curious to know whether or not a child has inherited it. In 1994, guidelines were issued by the UK Clinical Genetics Society about predictive genetic testing in children [21]. These and other subsequent national and international guidelines recommend that, where there is no anticipated medical benefit (e.g. preventative or therapeutic actions that could be initiated), testing should be deferred until such time there was, or the child is old enough to make an autonomous decision [22].

Much has been written about the potential psychosocial consequences of testing in the absence of medical benefit and the ethical issues involved [23, 24]. Most of the guidelines base their conclusions on the need to protect children's best interests, and that these are not served if there is no medical benefit to the testing. On the other hand, the debate has acknowledged both potential benefits of testing in childhood and psychological harms of not testing [25]. There may be wider best interests at stake other than medical ones and clinicians are not necessarily best placed to judge these. As the Genetic Interest Group put it in response to the UK guidelines: "Parents are responsible for welfare of children and at the end of the day most are better equipped to decide what is in the best interests of their child and family than outsiders are" [26].

Because of the existence of guidelines discouraging testing in childhood, there is little empirical evidence about the consequences of such testing and research is needed to know whether current guidelines are too cautious. In the meantime, where requests are made, clinicians should engage in discussions with parents about what the advantages and disadvantages of testing in childhood might be and whether or not it could be deferred until an age at which the child can take part in the consenting process. Where the onset of a condition is imminent and where an intervention is available (e.g. MEN, see Case history 2), there might be a different decision than if this is not the case (e.g. Li-Fraumeni syndrome) (see Table 6).

Table 6. Predictive genetic testing for cancer predisposition in childhood.

There are a variety of cancer syndromes for which predictive genetic testing is possible. The decision on whether or not and when to test may depend on which of three broad groups the disease in question falls into:

(a) Conditions for which medical interventions are available but onset not until adulthood (for example, hereditary breast or bowel disease; BRCA1/BRCA2 or hereditary non-polyposis colorectal cancer [HNPCC or Lynch syndrome]).

(b) Conditions for which medical interventions are available and onset is in childhood, but testing is requested well before the average age of onset (for example, familial adenomatous polyposis [FAP] or von Hippel-Lindau disease [VHL]).

(c) Conditions which may have childhood onset but for which there are no proven clinical interventions (for example, Li-Fraumeni syndrome [LFS]).

Prenatal and pre-implantation genetic diagnosis

Prenatal diagnosis determines whether or not a fetus has inherited the cancer predisposition in question. Although termination of pregnancy is clearly not an inevitable consequence of such testing, the possibility of this is usually the reason for testing at this stage. If a termination was not sought then a child could be born whose adult predisposition to cancer was already known, yet as noted above, interventions are unlikely during childhood and thus testing should ideally be deferred until they are adults. Whilst some would be optimistic about the likelihood of improved management and treatments before a child tested now reaches adulthood, in other cases the burden of disease in the family is so large that termination of affected pregnancies is contemplated (see Case history 3; Table 7).

Table 7. Prenatal diagnosis.

Case history 3

Katy in Case history 1, has been shown to have inherited the Lynch syndrome mutation present in her family. She underwent two-yearly colonoscopy and is well at the age of 30. At the antenatal booking appointment in her first pregnancy, her midwife tells her that if she wants a genetic test on her baby for Lynch syndrome she has a choice of chorionic villous samplng or amniocentesis to do so.

Katy had not thought about testing her pregnancy but assumes that it must be considered standard practice as she has been offered the test and is curious to know whether or not she has passed on the predisposition to cancer to her unborn child.

Katy's child will not be at risk of cancer for another 30 years or so; preventative and treatment options may improve in that time.

Learning points:

Explore issues such as prenatal diagnosis for adult onset diseases with great care and sensitivity. Do not offer as a routine test. If Katy has the test, but does not terminate an affected child, then a child will be born whose genetic predisposition as an adult is known, and this runs contrary to national and international guidelines. At the same time, in some families the burden of disease is so great that termination of pregnancy is considered.

An alternative to termination of pregnancy is the testing of an embryo before implantation (pre-implantation genetic diagnosis or PGD). Whilst the current technical limitations of this procedure mean that the chance of a successful pregnancy is much lower than with natural conception, it is preferable to some prospective parents because termination of an existing pregnancy can be avoided. In the UK, PGD requires a license from the Human Fertilisation and Embryology Authority (HFEA). Initial licenses were for fully (or almost fully) penetrant diseases such as cystic fibrosis and Huntington's disease. However, following a public consultation on what its policy should be for late onset conditions that are incompletely penetrant, the HFEA has recommended that it would be appropriate, in principle, to extend the use of PGD for cancer genes "because the features of the conditions are not incompatible with them being regarded as serious genetic conditions" (http://www.hfea.gov.uk/). However, concern has also been expressed about the lower penetrance of some cancer predispositions and hence the fact that cancer may never arise in mutation carriers.

Genetic information and discrimination

There has been much public debate about the potential for genetic information to cause discrimination, for example, by insurance or employment agencies. The UK Human Genetics Commission has recently called for comprehensive legal protection against "discrimination on any genetic grounds" (www.hgc.gov.uk). They noted that clinicians report that people are reluctant to take DNA tests that may be important for their health, because of fears that test results may be used to their disadvantage by third parties such as employers or insurance companies.

The UK insurance industry has a self-imposed moratorium, initially from 2001-2006 and then extended to 2011, that they will not ask policy holders to have a genetic test, or the results of a genetic test, for policies under £500,000 (life) and under £300,000 for other types. Above these limits, only tests approved by the Genetics and Insurance Commission (GAIC) (www.advisorybodies.doh.gov.uk/genetics/gaic/) can be used. To date this has only been approved for Huntington's disease.

However, family history of disease continues to be used to load or refuse premiums with much variation between companies in the sophistication of family history analysis.

Where to go for help

Most clinical genetics departments will have some facility for discussion of complex cases, either within their own department or in their local hospital through for example, a clinical ethics committee (www.ethics-network.org.uk/). The UK Genethics Club (www.genethicsclub.org) holds national meetings three times per year for discussion of ethical cases or issues. The Genethics Club aims to provide a forum for health professionals to explore ethical dilemmas or problems and works towards shared models of good practice [27].

Key points

♦ The ethical and legal aspects of inherited cancer syndromes are complex and evolving.

♦ Family history is an essential component of genetic diagnosis.

♦ Investigation of one family member may involve recording information about others and identifying them as being at risk, without their knowledge.

♦ Managing such families may raise issues of confidentiality and the approach to at-risk individuals who have not sought medical advice themselves.

♦ The approach to genetic testing of children depends on the natural history of the particular condition involved.

References

1. *Alternative approaches to bioethics.* Ashcroft R, Parker M, Widershoven G, Verkerk M, Lucassen AM, Eds. Cambridge: Cambridge University Press, 2005. ISBN 13: 9780521543156.
2. Tyler E, Lucassen A. 1 in 5 cancer risk assessments change on follow-up of family history information. Personal communication, July 2008.
3. Consent and confidentiality in genetic practice: guidance on genetic testing and sharing genetic information. A report of the Joint Committee on Medical Genetics, July 2006. Accessed from http://www.rcplondon.ac.uk/pubs/books/ccgp/, May 2008.
4. Lucassen A, Parker M, Wheeler R. Implications of data protection legislation for family history. *BMJ* 2006; 332: 299-301.
5. Lucassen A, Parker M. Revealing false paternity: some ethical considerations. *Lancet* 2001; 357: 1033-5.
6. Lucassen AM, Parker M, Wheeler R. Role of next of kin in accessing health records of deceased relatives. *BMJ* 2004; 328: 952-3.
7. General Medical Council. Duties of a doctor. London: GMC, 2000.
8. W v Egdell, 1 All ER 855, 1990.
9. Lucassen A, Parker M. Confidentiality and serious harm in genetics - preserving the confidentiality of one patient and preventing harm to relatives. *Eur J Hum Genet* 2004; 12: 93-7.
10. Human Genetics Commission. Inside information: balancing interests in the use of personal genetic data. London: HGC, 2002.
11. Davey A, Newson A, O'Leary P. Communication of genetic information within families: the case for familial comity. *J Bioeth Inq* 2006; 3: 161-6.
12. Lucassen A. Should families own genetic information? *BMJ* 2007; 335: 22.
13. Parker M, Lucassen A. Genetic information: a joint account? *BMJ*; 329: 165-7.
14. Claes E, Evers-Kiebooms G, Boogaerts A, *et al.* Communication with close and distant relatives in the context of genetic testing for hereditary breast and ovarian cancer in cancer patients. *Am J Med Genet* 2003; 116A: 11-9.
15. Clarke A, Richards M, Kerzin-Storrar L, *et al.* Genetic professionals' reports of nondisclosure of genetic risk information within families. *Eur J Hum Genet* 2005; 13: 556-62.
16. Pate v Threlkel, 661 So2d. 278 (FL, 1995).
17. Safer v Pack, 677 A.2d 1188, 683 A 2d 1163 (NJ, 1996).
18. Suthers GK, Armstrong J, McCormack J, Trott D. Letting the family know: balancing ethics and effectiveness when notifying relatives about genetic testing for a familial disorder. *J Med Genet* 2006; 43: 665-70.
19. Aktan-Collan K, Haukkala A, Pylvänäinen K, *et al.* Direct contact in inviting high-risk members of hereditary colon cancer families to genetic counselling and DNA testing. *J Med Genet* 2007; 44: 732-8.
20. Gilbar R. *The status of the family in law and bioethics: the genetic context.* Aldershot: Ashgate, 2005.

21. Clarke A. The genetic testing of children. Working party of the Clinical Genetics Society (UK). *J Med Genet* 2004; 31: 785-97.

22. Borry P, Stultiens L, Nys H, *et al.* Presymptomatic and predictive genetic testing in minors: a systematic review of guidelines and position papers. *Clinical Genetics* 2006; 70: 374-81.

23. Pelias MK. Genetic testing of children for adult-onset diseases: is testing in the child's best interests? *The Mount Sinai Journal of Medicine* 2006; 73: 605-8.

24. Michie S, Bowbrow M, Marteau TM on behalf of the FAP Collaborative Research Group. Predictive genetic testing in children and adults: a study of emotional impact. *J Med Genet* 2001; 38: 519-26.

25. Duncan RE, Savulescu J, Gillam L, *et al.* An international survey of predictive genetic testing in children for adult onset conditions. *Genet Med* 2005; 7: 390-6.

26. GIG response to the Clinical Genetics Society report: the genetic testing of children, 1995. Accessed May 08 from: www.gig.org.uk/docs/gig_testingchildren.pdf.

27. Lucassen AM, Parker M. The UK Genethics Club. *Clinical Ethics* 2006; 1: 219-23.

Chapter 4

Familial adenomatous polyposis

Sue Clark MD FRCS (Gen Surg)
Consultant Colorectal Surgeon and Assistant Director
The Polyposis Registry, St Mark's Hospital, Harrow, UK

Background

Patients with large numbers of adenomatous polyps in the colon and rectum were first documented in the late nineteenth century. As more and more cases were described it became clear that, at least in some, this clinical syndrome was inherited. Familial adenomatous polyposis (FAP) came to be defined by the presence of over 100 colorectal adenomas in an individual. Patients and their families were collected together by interested clinicians, notably Lockhart Mummery and Dukes at St Mark's Hospital in London [1]. The autosomal dominant inheritance pattern was confirmed and other clinical features were described. Surveillance of at-risk family members was developed and in the late 1940s, prophylactic surgery was introduced to prevent the development of colorectal cancer.

Over the next 30 years there were further refinements in the clinical management and follow-up. The genetic basis for the condition was identified as being located on the long arm of chromosome 5 by Bodmer [2] who identified an abnormality in this chromosome in a patient with FAP and mental retardation. Linkage studies later led to the identification of the responsible gene as being *APC* situated on 5q21 [3, 4], allowing genetic diagnosis and predictive genetic testing in many families.

Genetics

FAP is an autosomal dominantly inherited condition with almost 100% penetrance. An example of a pedigree originally described in 1925 and updated in 1973 is shown in Figure 1. In up to 85% of patients with a clinical phenotype of FAP, a mutation can be identified in the *APC* gene. These mutations almost all lead to the formation of a truncated protein product. The APC protein is a large and complex molecule that plays a key role in the wnt signalling pathway which is involved in cell division, differentiation and migration. It also has a role in mitotic spindle formation at cell division, as well as having a number of other potential functions. Mutation of the *APC* gene has been described as an early event in the formation of sporadic colorectal adenomas [5] and carcinomas. Thus, patients who inherit such mutations have 'taken the first step' towards colorectal adenoma formation from the moment they are conceived.

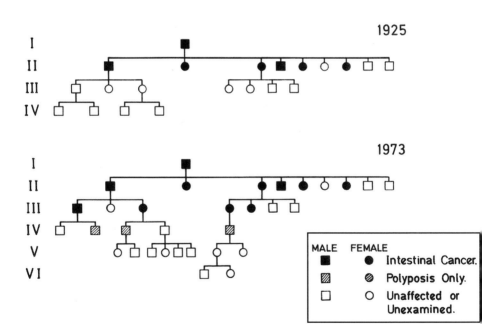

Figure 1. Pedigree of a family with FAP.

APC is a large gene and mutations have been described along almost its entire length. There are some common mutational hotspots (forming the 'mutation cluster region'). There is also evidence of 'genotype-phenotype correlation' in which the position of the mutation on the gene determines to some extent the clinical features manifested by the patient [6].

Each child of an affected individual carries a 50% chance of inheriting the mutated gene. In addition, about 20% of cases of FAP are due to a new mutation, the individual concerned having parents with no *APC* mutation.

APC gene mutation is thought to occur in about 1 in 10,000 of the population and this rate is constant throughout the different ethnic groups and geographical region studied to date. There is no gender difference.

Mouse model

A mouse model of FAP, the Min-mouse, which has a mutation in the mouse homologue of the *APC* gene (*Apc*), was serendipitously discovered in experiments using carcinogens to create mutations. These mice developed large numbers of adenomas in the small intestine, but did not tend to live long enough to develop invasive carcinoma. Experiments with these mice have shown that homozygous inheritance of a mutated *Apc* gene is incompatible with life.

A number of other models have been created using DNA technology to create specific mutations in the *Apc* gene.

Clinical picture

Large bowel

Until recently the presence of over 100 large bowel adenomas was considered pathognomonic of FAP. However, some patients with the recently described *MYH*-associated polyposis (MAP) (see Chapter 5) do have over a 100 adenomas.

The adenomas generally appear in late childhood and, unless prophylactic surgery is performed, will inevitably develop into colorectal cancer by the fourth or fifth decade of life [7]. The polyps are predominantly on the left side of the colon and in the rectum (Figure 2). They may number up to many thousands, carpeting the mucosa of the large bowel and sometimes resulting in anaemia, frank rectal bleeding or changes in bowel habit. Usually, affected individuals remain asymptomatic until the adenoma burden is very heavy or carcinoma develops.

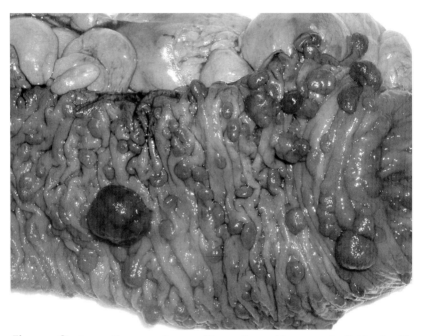

Figure 2. Operative specimen of large bowel from an individual with FAP.

Disease severity

Occasional individuals have been reported with an earlier onset of disease and presentation in childhood with symptoms. The earliest carcinoma described was in a five-year-old. Conversely, some individuals develop polyps much later in life and may never develop as many as 100. The term attenuated FAP (AFAP) has been coined to describe these families and certain mutations at the far ends of the gene have been found to correlate strongly with this milder phenotype [8]. Families with this variety of FAP do consistently tend to have a milder form of the disease. There is, however, also marked variation in polyp number and age of onset, and the presence and severity of extra-intestinal manifestations between members of the same family. This is thought to be due to the influence of modifier genes and environmental factors [6]. It can also often be difficult to determine or precisely define a phenotype, as much depends on the age of the individual concerned. For example, many will have prophylactic surgery before they develop as many adenomatous polyps as they would if the large bowel had been left intact.

Upper gastrointestinal tract

Ninety percent of patients with FAP will develop adenomatous polyps in the duodenum, particularly the ampullary region [9]. Overall, only about 10% progress to invasive carcinoma and this tends to occur at a later age than colorectal cancer. It does, however, carry an extremely poor prognosis.

Quite florid polyposis can sometimes be seen in the stomach, although biopsies show that this consists of cystic gland polyps which are not pre-malignant. There have been isolated reports of an increase in incidence of adenocarcinoma of the stomach in FAP, but these come from countries such as Japan and Korea where the background rate of gastric carcinoma is high.

There have been a handful of reports of jejunal and ileal carcinoma in FAP, but polyps at these sites are extremely uncommon in pre-operative patients. Adenomas, and even some carcinomas, seem to occur when the small bowel is exposed to faecal stasis, for example in ileo-anal pouches [10], in continent ileostomy (Kock) pouches and on ileostomy spouts.

Desmoid disease

Desmoids are extremely uncommon mesenchymal tumours that are locally invasive but do not metastasise. In FAP, they are over a thousand times more common than in the general population [11]. The underlying aetiology is not understood but their development is related in many cases to trauma (which is usually surgical), female gender and certain germline *APC* mutations.

Desmoids can occur anywhere in the body but in FAP they are most common within the abdomen. They also typically occur in the abdominal wall and in the para-spinous muscles (Figure 3). Outside the abdomen they can be troublesome because of their bulk, but within the abdomen can cause serious morbidity. They typically form in the small bowel mesentery where they cause compression and obstruction of the small bowel which can result in perforation. They may also obstruct the ureters, or compress great vessels and nerves causing venous thrombosis and pain.

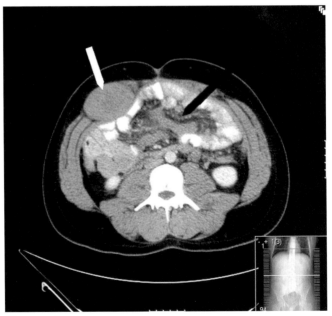

Figure 3. CT scan showing both abdominal wall (white arrow) and intra-abdominal (black arrow) desmoid.

Desmoids display unpredictable behaviour. Approximately 10% appear and then resolve spontaneously. A further 10% grow relentlessly and result ultimately in death. The remaining 80% tend to display stable or cyclical behaviour and while generally not fatal, cause considerable morbidity.

Other manifestations

Individuals with FAP have one mutated copy of the *APC* gene in every cell in the body. This results in a range of manifestations.

Many children with FAP develop supernumerary teeth. Benign osteomas, particularly of the mandible, are very common. Patients with FAP may develop epidermoid cysts at an early age (even in childhood) and at multiple sites. The term Gardner's syndrome was historically used to describe the co-existence of FAP, epidermoid cysts, desmoids and osteomas.

A number of otherwise rare malignancies are more common in FAP. These include hepatoblastoma, a form of papillary thyroid carcinoma and medulloblastoma.

Congenital hypertrophy of the retinal pigment epithelium (CHRPE) is a congenital pigmentation of the retina with a freckle-like appearance. Again, this occurs in the general population but is more common in FAP, with multiple and bilateral CHRPEs being found in some families. These are harmless lesions, but they were the object of great interest prior to the identification of the *APC* gene, as they offered a potential tool for screening at-risk children. Their presence is associated with mutations in a specific part of the *APC* gene.

Increasing use of cross-sectional imaging has shown that there is an excess of incidentally discovered adrenal masses in patients with FAP. The majority of these turn out to be non-hyperfunctioning adrenal adenomas, but phaeochromocytoma and adenocarcinoma have been reported.

Diagnosis and surveillance

The difficult diagnosis

The key to the diagnosis of FAP is the identification of a classical phenotype of over 100 colorectal adenomas. Once this has been established, genetic testing in that individual will identify an *APC* mutation in up to 85% of cases. Difficulties arise when polyps are identified but are not carefully counted. The use of dye spray in colonoscopy can greatly aid polyp identification and will often result in a described attenuated phenotype being reassigned as a classical one. Both endoscopists and pathologists should be encouraged to estimate polyp numbers to determine whether more or fewer than 100 are present and whether carpeting polyposis or a colonic burden of over a 1,000 is present, as this may change management.

Undoubtedly there are conditions predisposing to adenoma formation which result in a phenotype with fewer polyps and a weaker inheritance pattern than FAP, but these are not currently fully understood. Whilst surveillance is probably indicated in these circumstances, it is likely to be less intensive than in FAP and endoscopic management may well be perfectly acceptable.

Investigation of families with an FAP-like phenotype but no identified *APC* mutation has already led to the discovery of *MYH*-associated polyposis and may in future lead to the elucidation of further distinct conditions, although these are inevitably going to turn out to be less common than FAP.

A very strong family history of colorectal cancer inherited in an autosomal dominant fashion, but in the absence of significant adenomatous polyps, should raise the possibility of the diagnosis of hereditary non-polyposis colorectal cancer.

The existence of a genotype-specific genuinely attenuated form of FAP [8] can also cause some confusion, although improvements in mutation screening should reduce this.

Registries

Once the clinical features of FAP and the inheritance pattern had been described, a number of polyposis registries were started around the world. The aim of these institutions was to confirm the diagnosis in the index case and then identify at-risk family members, who could then be informed about their level of risk and offered appropriate surveillance. Anyone found to carry the condition could be offered appropriate management which initially was often treatment of pre-existing carcinomas but more latterly became prophylactic surgery in adolescence to prevent carcinoma formation [12].

Prior to the introduction of prophylactic surgery, most patients with FAP died of colorectal carcinoma in their forties and fifties. Prevention of this using prophylactic surgery produced a cohort of patients with FAP living to greater maturity. It became clear that these patients had further difficulties, particularly with desmoid disease and peri-ampullary carcinoma [13]. Clinicians at the polyposis registries have developed screening and management strategies for upper gastrointestinal polyposis, and increasingly also for desmoid disease and other manifestations.

It has been shown that care of these families in established registries has improved their life expectancy considerably [7, 12], although this remains somewhat below the level of the normal population. This is achieved by thorough family assessment, surveillance and exhaustive follow-up.

Genetic testing

Once the genetic basis for FAP was identified, the mutations responsible were characterised in an ever increasing proportion of affected individuals (currently about 85%). Once the causative mutation has been identified in an individual with FAP, it is a straightforward matter to perform predictive genetic testing on at-risk relatives to determine whether or not they have inherited the family mutation. If they have not, they do not have an excess risk of colorectal cancer and can be discharged from follow-up. If they have been found to have inherited the mutation they can then be offered surveillance and prophylactic surgery. Many registries now work closely with their local genetics departments or have qualified genetic counsellors working within them to facilitate this service.

In some centres pre-implantation diagnosis is available. This is a form of *in vitro* fertilisation, in which a cell is taken from each embryo and tested for presence of the family *APC* mutation. Only embryos which are free of the mutation are then implanted.

Some families with a clear autosomal dominant inheritance pattern and a definite phenotype of hundreds of adenomatous polyps do not as yet have an identifiable mutation. Some of these may indeed harbour *APC* mutations which are difficult to detect, or more subtle epigenetic changes that are simply technically impossible to identify using current technologies. A proportion may well turn out to have mutations in other genes, a good example of this being the recently identified *MYH*-associated polyposis.

Clinical surveillance

Prior to the advent of genetic testing, all at-risk family members had to be followed up clinically. This approach is still required in the minority of families where no mutation has been identified. Polyps tend not to develop until late childhood and generally children at risk are spared invasive investigation or indeed any medical contact until they reach the age of about 12 to 14 years. However, there have been isolated cases of an earlier onset of disease and even carcinoma, all of which have presented with symptoms in childhood. Therefore, any child at risk of having inherited FAP should be investigated whatever their age if they become symptomatic.

Clinical surveillance regimens vary from unit to unit [14] but that used at St Mark's Hospital consists of annual flexible sigmoidoscopy from the age of 14 years. From the age of 20 full colonoscopy is performed instead of the flexible sigmoidoscopy every fifth year. It is very difficult to know at what age this screening can safely cease. Over 90% of individuals with FAP will have developed polyps by the age of 25 or 30 and therefore the more time that goes by without polyps appearing the less likely it is that the individual concerned has the condition. However, in view of the variation in phenotype within families and the existence of attenuated FAP, surveillance should certainly be continued to the age of 50.

Clinical management (Figure 4)

Large bowel

Once the diagnosis of FAP has been confirmed, the aim is to remove the polyp-bearing large bowel before carcinoma can develop [14]. Some patients, notably with FAP due to a new mutation or those in whom family follow-up and surveillance has failed, may present with a diagnosis of cancer. This needs to be treated as appropriate to the stage of disease, but if it is potentially curable the aim of surgery should also be to offer prophylaxis to prevent the development of further cancer.

Timing of surgery
As in most cases polyps do not develop until late childhood and early adolescence screening does not need to begin until this time [14]. Even after a diagnosis of FAP has been confirmed there is usually a low polyp burden in the late teens, and it is possible to continue annual colonoscopic surveillance until an appropriate time for surgery is reached. The aim is that the affected individual should be of sufficient maturity to take part in the decision making process and that the surgery should be timed to interfere as little as possible with their education or employment. Usually this results in surgery being performed during a vacation between the ages of 14 and 18. There currently appears to be no advantage in undertaking surgery earlier except in those exceptional cases where there are symptoms or a high polyp burden at a younger age.

The choice of operation
The choice of prophylactic operation has changed with time [15]. Before the late 1940s, it was rarely done at all because of the high risks of surgery and anaesthesia. From 1948 onwards, colectomy with ileorectal anastomosis (IRA) was performed. The only alternative was pan-proctocolectomy with a permanent end-ileostomy and most individuals wished to avoid this procedure.

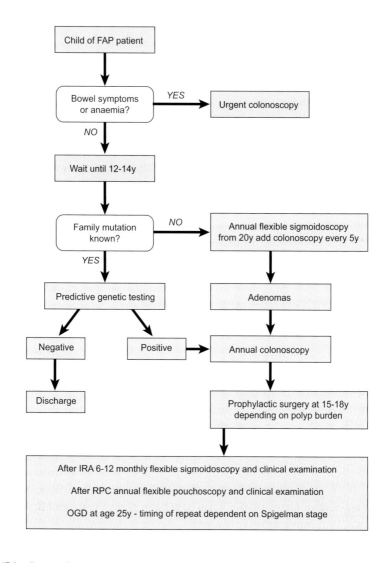

IRA = ileorectal anastomosis
RPC = restorative proctocolectomy
OGD = oesophago-gastro-duodenoscopy

Figure 4. Summary of management of an individual at risk of FAP.

IRA leaves the rectum in place. This part of the bowel can be relatively straightforwardly surveyed and polyps removed but it is essential that this is done regularly. Function is good and there is minimal morbidity associated with the operation.

Up until the late 1970s, surveillance was done using rigid sigmoidoscopy and polyps were removed with diathermy fulguration. Visualisation of the retained rectum was not ideal and the repeated fulguration caused dense rectal scarring increasing the difficulty of further surveillance. As time went by it became increasingly clear there was a significant incidence of cancer in the retained rectum associated with advancing age. Despite this the mortality rate from cancer occurring in the rectum after IRA remained low.

In the late 1970s, the restorative proctocolectomy (RPC) or ileo-anal pouch was described and offered the opportunity to remove all or virtually all of the at-risk large bowel mucosa. There is controversy as to whether a mucosectomy and hand-sewn anastomosis should be performed to remove the very lower most centimetre or so of mucosa.

Initially this procedure was greeted with great enthusiasm but recently it has become clear that there are several drawbacks. Bowel function (i.e. frequency and leakage) is not as good as following an IRA, an important issue when considering prophylactic surgery in an otherwise well adolescent. The morbidity and mortality associated with the procedure is higher and if the pouch fails, as ultimately approximately 10% do, a permanent end-ileostomy is required. Damage to the pelvic nerves at proctectomy carries a small (1-5%) risk of impotence or ejaculatory failure in men, and female fertility is approximately halved following the procedure. It was originally hoped that patients after RPC would not require any further follow-up but it has now been shown that most develop adenomas and, rarely, even carcinomas, in their pouches, some of which have to be removed.

RPC is therefore not the ideal prophylactic procedure and the current recommendation is that it be reserved for cases where there is a high risk of rectal cancer development if an IRA is performed [16]. These include: severe colorectal disease either in terms of existing phenotype (over 1000 colonic adenomas or over 20 rectal adenomas); a genotype which predicts a severe phenotype (codon 1309 mutation); when a patient presents with a rectal carcinoma; or at an age over 25 years. Recent evidence looking at retrospective data has shown that if these criteria are applied there is a very low risk of developing or dying from a rectal cancer in those who have an IRA. If rectal polyp burden does become an issue it is feasible to convert an IRA to an ileo-anal pouch (a restorative proctectomy) with no compromise with regard to morbidity, mortality or function, with the exception of the occasional case where a desmoid tumour makes this technically impossible.

Follow-up
After IRA, flexible sigmoidoscopy should be performed every six months to one year and polyps over 5mm should be removed. After RPC, annual pouchoscopy with removal of large polyps is recommended [14].

Chemoprevention
There is evidence that non-steroidal anti-inflammatories (NSAIDs) and COX-2 inhibitors [17] can decrease adenoma size and number in the large bowel. How much this impacts on cancer development is not known, and these drugs should certainly not be considered as treatment for FAP, even though they are licensed for use in this context. They may have a place in circumstances where the presence of a desmoid tumour or other comorbidity makes excision of the colon or rectum hazardous or even impossible.

Upper gastrointestinal tract

Surveillance
Upper gastrointestinal polyposis and cancer occur at a later age than the large bowel manifestations of FAP. Surveillance can therefore start later, at around the age of 25. Both forward and side-viewing scopes should be used to visualise the duodenum and ampullary area in detail. The Spigelman staging (Table 1) uses polyp size, number and histopathological features to quantify the severity of duodenal polyposis and follow-up intervals are determined according to this. Patients with mild disease are very unlikely to develop invasive carcinoma but those with stage IV duodenal polyposis are at 36% risk of developing an invasive carcinoma within the next ten years [18]. Once an invasive carcinoma develops the prognosis is very poor.

Table 1. Spigelman staging of duodenal adenomas in FAP.

No of polyps	Size of polyps (mm)	Histology	Dysplasia	Points
1 - 4	1 - 4	Tubular	Mild	1
5 - 20	5 - 10	Tubulovillous	Moderate	2
>20	>10	Villous	Severe	3

Total points	Spigelman stage	Interval to next duodenoscopy
0	0	5 years
1 - 4	I	5 years
5 - 6	II	3 years
7 - 8	III	1 year
9 - 12	IV	6 months

Management

Stage I and II disease can simply be watched. At stage III disease, the aim is endoscopic control using polypectomy, argon plasma coagulation and hot biopsy. Consideration can be given to introducing chemoprevention and there is some evidence that the COX-2 inhibitor, celecoxib, may reduce duodenal polyp burden to some extent [19].

Once stage IV is reached serious consideration should be given to prophylactic duodenectomy [18]. Despite the considerable mortality and morbidity of this procedure, the high risk of dying of invasive peri-ampullary or duodenal carcinoma if it is not performed justifies this aggressive approach in many cases.

Desmoid disease

There is very little evidence on which to base treatment for desmoid tumours [11]. Extra-abdominal and abdominal wall desmoids can be treated safely by surgery although recurrence rates are high. Those within the abdomen may be very hazardous to remove surgically, usually because of their close proximity to the superior mesenteric vessels. Historical series have documented high levels of morbidity and mortality following surgery for intra-abdominal desmoids, but more recently better results have been obtained, probably due to careful selection using high quality cross-sectional imaging. In a few circumstances patients have required a total enterectomy followed by either lifelong total parenteral nutrition or even small bowel transplantation.

Ureteric obstruction should be treated by stenting, and obstructed or perforated bowel may be best managed by laparotomy and proximal diversion without an attempt to excise the desmoid.

There have been several small uncontrolled series which have reported good results treating desmoids with NSAIDs (principally sulindac) and also with anti-oestrogens (tamoxifen and toremifene). The variable natural history of desmoids makes interpretation of these difficult. Some groups have used cytotoxic chemotherapy (doxorubicin and dacarbazine or vinblastine and methotrexate) in relentlessly progressive desmoids with good results, but this type of treatment with its potential adverse effects should be avoided in all but the most severe disease.

Prediction of aggressive disease and successful treatment remain major challenges.

Other manifestations

Most of the other manifestations of FAP are either entirely benign, such as epidermoid cysts which can be excised in the usual way, or are unusual cancers which should be treated in the same way as those occurring sporadically. Occasionally identification of an unusual cancer or a desmoid tumour in a young patient might raise the suspicion of FAP and trigger investigation of the large bowel and diagnosis.

The future

The main challenges for the future care of patients with FAP centre on ensuring a continuation of high quality family screening and surveillance with appropriate access to genetic services.

A research focus on families where no mutation has so far been identified, coupled with improvements in technology should clarify the genetic diagnosis in most cases. In some cases this will be due to more sensitive *APC* gene mutation detection, and in others to the identification of other genes resulting in a similar clinical picture.

Advances in chemoprevention might delay the age at which prophylactic surgery is required or conceivably in future abolish it altogether, although this currently seems a distant prospect. Pre-implantation diagnosis may well reduce the number of children born to families with FAP who inherit the disease but the occurrence of new mutations will mean that there will continue to be new cases of FAP diagnosed.

Duodenal and peri-ampullary carcinoma and desmoid disease are major FAP-related causes of morbidity and mortality. Both present enormous challenges, particularly in terms of identifying the minority with serious disease early, and then in providing effective treatment.

Key points

◆ FAP is an autosomal dominantly inherited syndrome with almost 100% penetrance for colorectal adenomas and cancer.

◆ Without prophylactic surgery virtually all patients with FAP die before the age of 50 years from colorectal cancer.

◆ Most adenomatous colorectal polyps develop in adolescence, and colectomy or proctocolectomy is recommended by the late teens to prevent cancer development.

◆ There are a number of other manifestations of the disease, and upper gastrointestinal cancer and desmoid disease have become significant problems now that patients with FAP are living longer.

◆ Systematic and organised care of patients with FAP and their families is best provided through dedicated polyposis registries (Figure 4).

References

1. Dukes C. The hereditary factor in polyposis intestine, or multiple adenomata. *Cancer Review* 1930; 5: 241-51.

2. Bodmer WF, Bailey CJ, Bodmer J, *et al*. Localisation of the gene for familial adenomatous polyposis on chromosome 5. *Nature* 1987; 328: 614-6.

3. Kinzler KW, Nilbert MC, Su LK, *et al*. Identification of FAP locus genes from chromosome 5q21. *Science* 1991; 253: 661-5.

4. Groden J, Thliveris A, Samowitz W, *et al*. Identification and characterization of the familial adenomatous polyposis coli gene. *Cell* 1991; 66: 589-600.

5. Fodde R. The *APC* gene in colorectal cancer. *Eur J Cancer* 2002; 20: 905-11.

6. Crabtree MD, Tomlinson IPM, Hodgson SV, *et al*. Explaining variation in familial adenomatous polyposis: relationship between genotype and phenotype and evidence for modifier genes. *Gut* 2002; 51: 420-3.

7. Nugent KP, Spigelman AD, Phillips RKS. Life expectancy after colectomy and ileorectal anastomosis for familial adenomatous polyposis. *Dis Colon Rectum* 1993; 36: 1059-62.

8. Hernegger GS, Moore HG, Guillem JG. Attenuated familial adenomatous polyposis: an evolving and poorly understood entity. *Dis Colon Rectum* 2002; 45: 127-34.

9. Wallace MH, Phillips RKS. Upper gastrointestinal disease in patients with familial adenomatous polyposis. *Br J Surg* 1998; 85: 742-50.

10. Groves CJ, Beveridge G, Swain DJ, *et al*. Prevalence and morphology of pouch and ileal adenomas in familial adenomatous polyposis. *Dis Colon Rectum* 2005; 48: 816-23.

11. Sturt NJH, Clark SK. Current ideas in desmoid tumours. *Familial Cancer* 2006; 5: 275-85.

12. Bulow S. Results of national registration of familial adenomatous polyposis. *Gut* 2003; 52: 742-6.

13. Belchez LA, Berk T, Bapat BV, *et al*. Changing causes of mortality in patients with familial adenomatous polyposis. *Dis Colon Rectum* 1996; 9: 384-7.

14. Church J, Simmang C. Practice parameters for the treatment of patients with dominantly inherited colorectal cancer (familial adenomatous polyposis and hereditary nonpolyposis colorectal cancer). *Dis Colon Rectum* 2003; 46: 1001-12.

15. Church J, Burke C, McGannon E, *et al*. Risk of rectal cancer after colectomy and ileorectal anastomosis for familial adenomatous polyposis: a function of available options. *Dis Colon Rectum* 2003; 46: 1175-81.

16. Bulow C, Vasen H, Jarvinen H, *et al*. Ileorectal anastomosis is appropriate for a subset of patients with familial adenomatous polyposis. *Gastroenterology* 2000; 119: 1454-60.

17. Steinbach LT, Lynch P, Phillips RKS, *et al*. The effect of celecoxib, a cyclo-oxygenase inhibitor, in familial adenomatous polyposis. *New Engl J Med* 2000; 342: 1946-58.

18. Groves CJ, Saunders BP, Spigelman AD, Phillips RKS. Duodenal cancer in patients with familial adenomatous polyposis (FAP): results of a 10-year prospective study. *Gut* 2002; 50: 636-41.

19. Phillips RKS, Wallace MH, Lynch PM, *et al*. A randomised, double blind, placebo controlled study of celecoxib, a selective cyclo-oxygenase 2 inhibitor, on duodenal polyposis in familial adenomatous polyposis. *Gut* 2002; 50: 857-60.

Chapter 5

MYH-associated polyposis

Olivia Will MB ChB MRCS(Eng)
Surgical Research Fellow
The Polyposis Registry, St Mark's Hospital, Harrow, UK

Background

The mutY human homologue (*MYH*) gene is the most recently discovered cause of colonic adenomatous polyposis, identified in 2002. Its discovery was suggested by three observations. Firstly, despite sophisticated laboratory techniques, a germline *APC* mutation could not be identified in some patients with the clinical phenotype of familial adenomatous polyposis. Secondly, some patients with adenomatous polyposis had a family pedigree suggesting autosomal recessive, rather than dominant inheritance (Figure 1). Lastly, the polyps from these patients showed an unusual pattern of acquired mutations [1].

Genetics

MYH is located on chromosome 1p, and is one of three identified genes involved in base-excision-repair (BER), the others being *OGG1* and *MTH* [1]. BER proteins (like mismatch repair proteins) ensure genomic integrity by repairing damage before replication, thus preventing transmission of mutations to progeny cells. Whereas Lynch syndrome can be due to mutation of any one of a number of mismatch repair genes, only mutation of *MYH* has been shown to cause disease [2, 3], now known as *MYH*-associated polyposis, or MAP.

A guide to cancer genetics in clinical practice

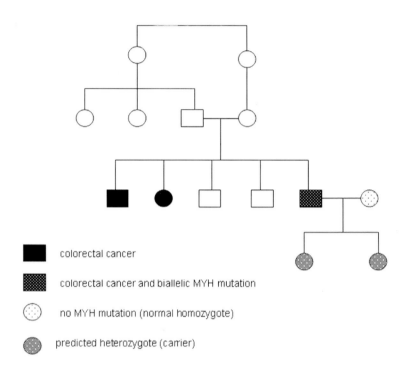

■ colorectal cancer

▨ colorectal cancer and biallelic MYH mutation

⊙ no MYH mutation (normal homozygote)

● predicted heterozygote (carrier)

Figure 1. Pedigree of a family with MAP arising following the marriage of first cousins.

BER proteins are glycosylases that repair oxidative damage of DNA [4]. In normal DNA, G pairs with C, and A with T. However, oxidised guanine results in incorrect oxoG-T pairing in the DNA strand. In subsequent replication, the error is compounded by A-T pairing in the strand replicated from the incorrectly paired base. Effectively, this results in a GC:TA mutation. This was the characteristic somatic mutation found in colonic tumours in patients, which led to the identification of the faulty BER gene as a cause of colonic tumourigenesis. Frequently, this transversion occurs in the *APC* gene [5], and it is therefore not surprising that MAP shares many features with FAP; in both cases, the end result is *APC* inactivation in colonocytes.

In important respects, however, MAP differs from other inherited causes of colorectal cancer. Unlike sporadic and FAP-associated tumours, which show a high degree of chromosomal instability, MAP tumours were found to be near diploid, and yet are also without the features of microsatellite instability common in Lynch syndrome. Thus, MAP tumours appear to follow a distinct genetic pathway [6], a molecular finding which may influence tumour behaviour, and may have implications for future chemotherapeutics.

Clinical picture

Table 1 highlights the major phenotypic differences between MAP, FAP and Lynch syndrome.

Table 1. Comparison between clinical characteristics of FAP, Lynch syndrome (LS) and MAP.

	FAP	LS	MAP
Colonic polyps	Typically 1000s	Typically scanty	Very variable
Upper GI polyps	Often numerous	None	Sometimes
Skin/mesodermal manifestations	Epidermoid cysts, osteomas, CHRPE, desmoids, dental abnormalities	Café-au-lait macules in homozygotes	As yet undetermined
Common extra-colonic cancers	Duodenal cancer hepatoblastoma	Endometrium, urothelium, ovary, stomach, brain,	Breast cancer?
Average age of colorectal cancer	40	50	50
Heterozygous risk of colorectal cancer	100%	70%	Low (homozygous risk may be nearly 100%)
Population incidence of heterozygotes	1:10,000	1:1000	1:100

Large bowel

It is a common misconception that MAP always causes less severe polyposis than FAP. Patients with MAP may have thousands of polyps, and thus one cannot distinguish between them in terms of polyp burden. Figure 2 demonstrates this point. Although there are contradictory findings in the literature, a large cohort study of 40 patients found that there was an equal likelihood of attenuated (<100 polyps) and classical polyposis phenotypes [5].

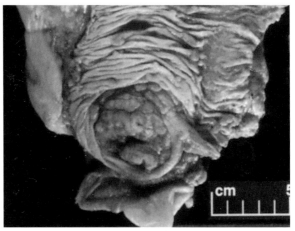

Figure 2. Colectomy specimen from a patient with MAP.

Biallelic mutation carriers may develop more right-sided cancers, at a slightly older age than FAP, around 47 years. Most studies have consistently found that patients with MAP are more likely than those with FAP to be diagnosed with colon cancer - perhaps due to improved screening of those identified to be at risk of FAP.

Long-term outcomes for MAP patients with colorectal cancer are yet to be determined. It is reasonable to assume that there may be a different response to chemotherapy in these patients due to the underlying defect in BER. Tumour behaviour in terms of rate of progression and metastasis may also differ in MAP. However, patient numbers are small and there are no published data to answer these important questions.

Upper gastrointestinal tract

Patients with MAP may also have fundic polyps and duodenal polyps, and duodenal, as well as gastric cancer, has been reported. However, the proportion of patients with upper gastrointestinal disease may be less than in FAP [7]; reports vary from about one in three to one in five patients having duodenal polyps.

Other manifestations

Breast cancer was found to occur in 18% of female biallelic mutation carriers [5]; this has yet to be confirmed in further studies. Thyroid cancer was reported in a single patient, and osteomas and dental cysts are also documented. Reports of skin manifestations include pilomatricomas, sebaceous gland tumours, and café-au-lait spots were noted in the St Mark's E466X patients (unpublished data). There are no reports of desmoid tumours in MAP.

Diagnosis and surveillance

Genetic testing

Estimations of prevalence and risk are in flux as more information gathers in the published literature on this recently characterised condition. Currently, it is thought that biallelic germline *MYH* mutations (usually compound heterozygote with a different mutation of each allele, but occasionally homozygote) cause approximately 0.4-3% of unselected colorectal cancers, and are usually associated with multiple adenomas; however, cases have been reported with extremely low polyp counts [8]. The autosomal recessive inheritance, and occasionally mild polyposis phenotype, means that MAP may frequently be undiagnosed in patients presenting with colorectal cancer.

MYH mutation screening is now available for patients with adenomatous polyposis, in whom germline *APC* screening failed to demonstrate a mutation, or in those with colorectal polyps or cancer in whom autosomal recessive inheritance is likely (consanguineous parentage or isolated geography). Immunohistochemistry of tumour specimens is also being developed [9], which will allow retrospective diagnosis in archival samples.

The population prevalence of heterozygotes is estimated at 1:100. Thus, when an individual is diagnosed as having MAP, mutation screening can be offered to his or her spouse, and first-degree relatives. This will allow estimation of risk to the offspring. The autosomal recessive pattern of inheritance poses challenges for a clinician or polyposis registry, since the extended family should be referred for assessment, in order to proactively identify people at risk. In relatives, the entire gene should be screened (rather than simply screening for the mutations found in the proband), since compound heterozygosity is common. For further identified heterozygotes, screening should be offered in turn for their spouses and children. Since the population incidence of heterozygotes is estimated to be 1:100, thorough case finding is likely to prove expensive. However, this is extremely important in cultural groups where consanguineous marriage is common.

Varying *MYH* mutations predominate in different populations: for example, studies of UK Caucasians show a preponderance of the Y165C and G382D mutations, while Y90X is more common in patients from Pakistan, E466X in Indians, and nt1395delGGA in those of Mediterranean origin. In this way, mutation screening is aided by focusing on the most likely candidates in turn, guided by the patient's ethnicity.

Cancer risk

The lifetime risk of developing colorectal cancer for a person homozygous (or compound heterozygous) for an *MYH* mutation is estimated at almost 100% at 60 years [10] - a very high penetrance, similar to that of FAP. The lifetime risk for a heterozygote is not yet fully determined, but current studies indicate that a mono-allelic carrier may have a small increased risk (1.6) of colorectal cancer compared to the general population [11], and this may be significant only in those older than 55 years. However, population-based studies are difficult in rare conditions, and in the mouse model $Apc^{(Min/+)}/Myh^{(+/-)}$, *Myh* heterozygosity conferred no increased risk of adenomas [12].

Genotype-phenotype correlations

In FAP, there is a strong genotype-phenotype correlation, with both intestinal and extra-intestinal manifestations varying according to the patient's inherited germline mutation. As yet, no similar correlation has been identified for the common *MYH* mutations. In addition, it seems that the homozygotes and compound heterozygotes have similar disease severity.

Clinical management

Affected individuals will develop cancer without treatment, so preventative measures need to be focused on the colon, upper gastrointestinal tract, and breasts in female patients. While treatment is not standardised between centres, the protocols presented here for intestinal surveillance are those currently used at St Mark's Hospital.

Large bowel

The colon should be assessed by dye-spray colonoscopy. Treatment should be tailored to the polyp burden. Large numbers of polyps, or a high degree of dysplasia on biopsy, indicate the need for prophylactic colectomy, as performed in FAP. There are no data regarding the benefit of pharmaceutical agents, such as COX-2 inhibitors, to decrease polyp burden in MAP.

Scanty polyps with low-grade dysplasia may be managed expectantly by regular colonoscopy [13], on a one or two-yearly basis, or as per current guidelines for sporadic polyps, whichever is more frequent. The first colonoscopy should be at the time of diagnosis or at age 25, since 95% of cancers occur after the age of 35 years. The decision to defer colectomy in those with mild disease rests on the supposition that cancer risk correlates directly with polyp burden. Patients need to be aware that there are no long-term follow-up data and that there remains a risk of developing cancer despite surveillance; in some cases, cancers may arise without visible adenomas. Some recommend colectomy for homozygotes irrespective of polyp burden for this reason [14].

Upper gastrointestinal tract

The stomach and duodenum should be examined by side-viewing gastroduodenoscopy, also starting at age 25. Intervals for further screening are currently based on Spigelman staging for duodenal disease in FAP: mild disease should be rechecked at five-yearly intervals, which may be increased to three-yearly or annual checks. Severe disease requires assessment for surgery, as in FAP.

Breasts

Breast screening should be considered in female patients; at the very least, while evidence regarding the role of breast cancer screening is not yet available, female patients should be made aware of the risks of breast cancer and advised to practise regular self-examination.

Carriers

Heterozygotes may have a marginally increased risk of colorectal cancer, probably from the age of 55. At St Mark's, patients are offered initial colonoscopy at diagnosis, with repeat colonoscopies five-yearly until age 80 or comorbidities outweigh the benefits of the procedure. Upper gastrointestinal endoscopy is not required.

The future

Current information of the epidemiology and natural history of MAP is limited by the fact that it was identified so recently. Identification of new cases and follow-up of those known to be affected will increase our knowledge of this condition and the heterozygous carrier state, allowing evidenced-base surveillance and management protocols to be developed.

Key points

♦ MAP is a rare condition, accounting for <3% of colorectal cancers overall.

♦ Inheritance is autosomal recessive and incidence is higher in populations where consanguineous marriage is common.

♦ MAP has many features in common with FAP, and cancer prevention in homozygotes requires similar surveillance and management.

♦ The population incidence of heterozygotes is high, and if an increased risk is confirmed in heterozygotes, this will place a significant burden on genetic and screening services.

♦ Much further research is required to refine our understanding and management of MAP.

References

1. Al-Tassan N, Chmiel NH, Maynard J, *et al.* Inherited variants of *MYH* associated with somatic G:C-->T:A mutations in colorectal tumors. *Nat Genet* 2002; 30: 227-32.

2. Halford SE, Rowan AJ, Lipton L, *et al.* Germline mutations but not somatic changes at the *MYH* locus contribute to the pathogenesis of unselected colorectal cancers. *Am J Pathol* 2003; 162: 1545-8.

3. Sieber OM, Lipton L, Crabtree M, *et al.* Multiple colorectal adenomas, classic adenomatous polyposis, and germ-line mutations in *MYH*. *N Engl J Med* 2003; 348: 791-9.

4. Russo MT, De Luca G, Degan P, Bignami M. Different DNA repair strategies to combat the threat from 8-oxoguanine. *Mutat Res* 2007; 614(1-2): 69-76.

5. Nielsen M, Franken PF, Reinards TH, *et al.* Multiplicity in polyp count and extracolonic manifestations in 40 Dutch patients with *MYH*-associated polyposis coli (MAP). *J Med Genet* 2005; 42: e54.

6. Lipton L, Halford SE, Johnson V, *et al.* Carcinogenesis in *MYH*-associated polyposis follows a distinct genetic pathway. *Cancer Res* 2003; 63: 7595-9.

7. Kanter-Smoler G, Bjork J, Fritzell K, *et al.* Novel findings in Swedish patients with *MYH*-associated polyposis: mutation detection and clinical characterization. *Clin Gastroenterol Hepatol* 2006; 4: 499-506.

8. Enholm S, Hienonen T, Suomalainen A, *et al.* Proportion and phenotype of *MYH*-associated colorectal neoplasia in a population-based series of Finnish colorectal cancer patients. *Am J Pathol* 2003; 163: 827-32.

9. Di Gregorio C, Frattini M, Maffei S, *et al.* Immunohistochemical expression of MYH protein can be used to identify patients with *MYH*-associated polyposis. *Gastroenterology* 2006; 131: 439-44.

10. Farrington SM, Tenesa A, Barnetson R, *et al.* Germline susceptibility to colorectal cancer due to base-excision repair gene defects. *Am J Hum Genet* 2005; 77: 112-9.

11. Tenesa A, Campbell H, Barnetson R, *et al.* Association of MUTYH and colorectal cancer. *Br J Cancer* 2006; 95: 239-42.

12. Sieber OM, Howarth KM, Thirlwell C, *et al.* Myh deficiency enhances intestinal tumorigenesis in multiple intestinal neoplasia (ApcMin/+) mice. *Cancer Res* 2004; 64: 8876-81.

13. Fornasarig M, Minisini AM, Viel A, *et al.* Twelve years of endoscopic surveillance in a family carrying biallelic Y165C *MYH* defect: report of a case. *Dis Colon Rectum* 2006; 49: 272-5.

14. Leite JS, Isidro G, Martins M, *et al.* Is prophylactic colectomy indicated in patients with *MYH*-associated polyposis? *Colorectal Dis* 2005; 7: 327-31.

Chapter 6

Lynch syndrome (hereditary non-polyposis colorectal cancer)

Huw Thomas MA PhD FRCP
Professor of Gastrointestinal Genetics and Consultant Gastroenterologist
Imperial College, St Mark's Hospital, Harrow, UK

Background

In 1913 Warthin described a family in which there appeared to be an inherited predisposition to the development of stomach, endometrial and colorectal cancers [1]. Lynch followed up this family and described additional families with an inherited predisposition to colorectal and other cancers in the 1960s [2]. In contrast to familial adenomatous polyposis and the recently described *MYH*-associated polyposis these families did not have multiple colorectal polyps. The condition was termed hereditary non-polyposis colorectal cancer (HNPCC) to emphasise the contrast to familial adenomatous polyposis.

In the early 1990s cancers from affected members from these families were found to have genetic alterations in the tumours that were characteristic of changes that have been described in bacteria and yeast with defective DNA mismatch repair. Mutations of two DNA mismatch repair (MMR) genes (*MLH1* and *MSH2*) were detected in two different families with HNPCC [3, 4] and subsequently alterations of two further DNA mismatch repair genes (*MSH6* and *PMS2*) were also described in other families [5, 6].

Much confusion surrounds the terminology in this area. Families with an inherited defect of DNA mismatch repair are now defined as Lynch syndrome. This is inherited in an autosomal dominant fashion and predictive genetic testing may be undertaken in affected families. There remains a proportion of families with a strong genetic predisposition to colorectal cancer who do not have an inherited defect of DNA mismatch repair and in whom the genetic defect has yet to be identified. These are now termed familial colorectal cancer families. The term HNPCC is used confusingly by some authors to cover familial colorectal cancer and Lynch syndrome, and by others as synonymous with Lynch syndrome.

Genetics

Lynch syndrome is an autosomal dominantly inherited condition with a high penetrance for the development of cancer (Figure 1). The condition is heterogeneous with alterations of one of four different DNA mismatch

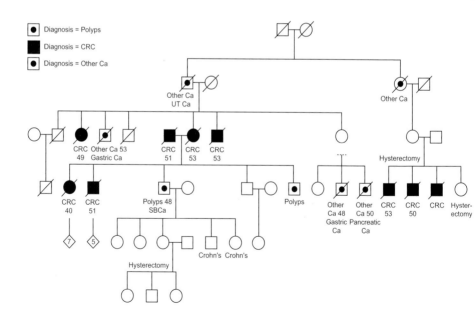

Figure 1. Pedigree of a family with Lynch syndrome. CRC=colorectal cancer; UT Ca=ureteric cancer.

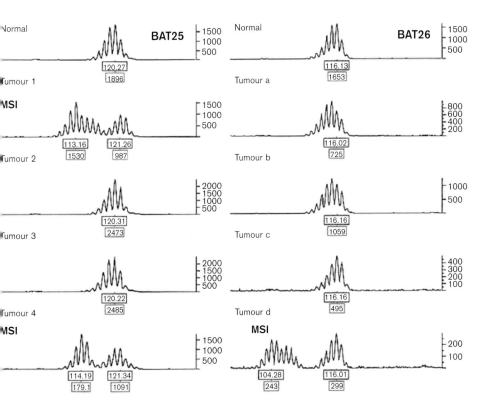

Figure 2. A trace of the PCR products of the microsatellite markers *BAT25* and *BAT26*. Additional peaks at *BAT25* in tumours 1 and 4 and at *BAT26* in tumour d indicate microsatellite instability (MSI) in these tumours.

repair genes being inherited in different families. These alterations lead to the inheritance of one normal copy of the gene and one altered copy of the gene. If a somatic mutation of the single normal copy of the gene occurs this causes defective DNA mismatch repair in an individual cell. Defective mismatch repair itself may lead to the accumulation of numerous mismatches in replicating DNA. The tumours from individuals with Lynch syndrome have a characteristic alteration of their DNA as a result of this which is known as microsatellite instability (Figure 2). These alterations may be detected quite simply in tumours and allow the identification of families that may have Lynch syndrome.

There is a 50% risk of the child of an affected individual with Lynch syndrome inheriting the mutated gene; there is no gender difference. A small proportion of Lynch syndrome patients may result from a new mutation.

Lynch syndrome is thought to account for approximately 2% of colorectal cancers, although founder mutations in some populations, such as in Finland [7], may lead to a higher proportion.

Approximately 15% of sporadic (non-familial) colorectal cancers also have defective colorectal mismatch repair with microsatellite instability. However, in these individuals the alteration results from an epigenetic change with methylation of the promoter of the *MLH1* DNA mismatch repair gene during tumourigenesis, which prevents gene transcription. This is not an inherited condition [8].

Clinical picture

Unlike familial adenomatous polyposis, Lynch syndrome does not have a characteristic clinical phenotype. The syndrome is associated with the development of colorectal, endometrial, ovarian, gastric, renal tract, brain, small bowel and bile duct cancers. The association of colorectal cancers and brain tumours has in the past been termed Turcot's syndrome. Affected individuals may also develop keratoacanthomas and sebaceous gland adenomas of the skin.

Colorectal cancer

The median age for the development of colorectal cancer in Lynch syndrome has been estimated at 44 years, although more recent population studies suggest that it may be older [9]. Colorectal cancers in Lynch syndrome are uncommon below the age of 25. A high proportion of the cancers are right-sided, occurring proximal to the splenic flexure, in contrast to sporadic colorectal cancers which are predominantly left-sided, occurring distal to the splenic flexure. There is evidence from the high incidence of interval cancers occurring during colonoscopic surveillance that colorectal cancers in Lynch syndrome develop more rapidly than sporadic colorectal cancers, and it has been proposed that this may be due to defective mismatch repair resulting in the rapid accumulation of mutations. Synchronous colorectal cancers are also common. The lifetime risk of colorectal cancer in men has been estimated at between 28% and 75%, and in women between 24% and 52% [10].

Histology
Colorectal cancers in Lynch syndrome have characteristic histopathological features with tumour infiltrating lymphocytes, a Crohn's-like lymphocytic reaction, mucinous/signet-ring differentiation and medullary growth pattern [11].

Prognosis
Colorectal cancers in Lynch syndrome and sporadic colorectal cancers with mismatch repair deficiency appear to have an improved five-year survival in comparison with sporadic colorectal cancers of the same stage and may have a different response to some chemotherapy [12]. There is evidence that Lynch syndrome cancers and sporadic colorectal cancers with microsatellite instability are unresponsive to treatment with 5-fluorouracil (5FU). *In vitro* studies suggest that MMR-deficient colorectal cancer cells do not respond to 5FU-based chemotherapy and most clinical studies have demonstrated no benefit with 5FU treatment in microsatellite unstable colorectal cancers [13, 14].

Endometrial and ovarian cancer

Endometrial cancer is common in women with Lynch syndrome and may be particularly common in those who carry an *MSH6* mutation. The lifetime risk of endometrial cancer has been estimated to be between 27% and 71%, and that of ovarian cancer between 3% and 13%.

Other gastrointestinal tract cancers

There was a high instance of gastric cancer in the families originally described by Warthin [1], although the lifetime risk of gastric cancer now appears to be lower, and has been estimated at between 2% and 13%.

There is a greatly increased relative risk of small bowel cancer which is rare in the general population; the absolute lifetime risk has been estimated at between 4% and 7% in Lynch syndrome. Bile duct and gallbladder cancers are also more common with a lifetime risk of approximately 2%.

Skin tumours

A small proportion of individuals with Lynch syndrome have characteristic skin tumours with keratoacanthomas occurring particularly on some light exposed areas and sebaceous gland adenomas which are often particularly noticeable on the face. The association of skin tumours and colorectal cancer has previously been called Muir-Torre syndrome.

Diagnosis

Lynch syndrome is difficult to diagnose as there is not a characteristic phenotype. It requires a high degree of clinical suspicion, particularly in families where there is a strong history of colorectal and other Lynch syndrome-associated cancers or where colorectal and other cancers have occurred synchronously or at an early age. The Amsterdam and Bethesda criteria were created and modified to aid this process and may be used to select patients with an increased risk of Lynch syndrome in whom molecular genetic analysis should be undertaken.

The Amsterdam criteria II

These criteria (Table 1) [15] were developed to identify families that have a high likelihood of harbouring an autosomal dominantly inherited cancer predisposition. They were not intended to be diagnostic criteria.

Population-based studies of consecutive colorectal cancer cases indicate that approximately 2% are due to inherited mismatch repair gene defects. A study in Columbus, Ohio, identified 23 mutation carriers out of 1066 colorectal cancer cases. It is of note that ten of these cases were

Table 1. Amsterdam criteria II.
◆ There should be at least three relatives with colorectal cancer or a Lynch syndrome-associated cancer (endometrium, small bowel, ureter or renal pelvis).
◆ One relative should be a first-degree relative of the other two.
◆ At least two successive generations should be affected.
◆ At least one tumour should be diagnosed before the age of 50.
◆ FAP should be excluded in the colorectal cancer case, if any.
◆ Tumours should be verified by pathological examination.

greater than 50 years of age at diagnosis, only three cases were from families that fulfilled the Amsterdam criteria, and five cases did not fulfil either the Amsterdam or the Bethesda criteria [16]. Generally it appears that approximately 50% of families that fulfil the Amsterdam criteria have Lynch syndrome (the remainder having familial colorectal cancer, or representing chance clustering), and that only 50% of individuals with Lynch syndrome come from families which fulfil them.

The revised Bethesda criteria

These criteria (Table 2) [17] define individuals with a diagnosis of colorectal cancer who are at increased risk of having Lynch syndrome, such that microsatellite instability or mismatch repair immunohistochemistry studies of their tumour should be performed.

Registries

Individuals with a strong family history of colorectal and/or Lynch syndrome-associated cancers fulfilling the Amsterdam criteria II should be referred to a regional genetic centre or a clinic with a particular interest in inherited cancer. Similarly, individuals with colorectal cancer who fulfil the revised Bethesda guidelines should have their tumours tested.

Table 2. Revised Bethesda criteria.

♦ Colorectal cancer diagnosed in the patient of less than 50 years of age.

♦ Presence of synchronous or metachronous colorectal or other Lynch syndrome-related tumours regardless of age.

♦ Colorectal cancer with histology suggestive of microsatellite instability diagnosed in a patient of less than 60 years of age.

♦ Patient with colorectal cancer and a first-degree relative with a Lynch syndrome-associated tumour with one cancer diagnosed under the age of 50 years.

♦ Patient with colorectal cancer with two or more first-degree relatives or second-degree relatives with a Lynch syndrome-related tumour regardless of age.

Lynch syndrome-related tumours include: colorectal, endometrial, stomach, ovarian, pancreas, ureter, renal pelvis, biliary tract, small bowel and brain cancers, sebaceous gland adenomas and keratoacanthomas.

The regional genetic clinic will verify the cancers that have occurred in the family and, if appropriate, undertake genetic testing of the tumour and subsequent germline mutation detection. The clinic will be able to ensure that at-risk family members are offered appropriate surveillance, and that at-risk family members are also able to discuss whether they wish to undergo predictive genetic testing.

Genetic analysis of tumours

In individuals from families that fulfil the Amsterdam criteria II or revised Bethesda guidelines, analysis of tumour tissue from an affected family member may be undertaken. Initially this may be by either immunohistochemistry or the detection of microsatellite instability. Mismatch repair genes are expressed in tissue and the protein product may be detected by immunohistochemistry. If in addition to the inherited alteration of the gene there is a somatic mutation of the normal copy in a tumour, this often leads to absence of the protein and loss of expression on immunohistochemistry. Alternatively, the tumour may be analysed for the presence of microsatellite instability using a panel of microsatellite primers in a PCR reaction.

As noted above, up to 15% of sporadic colorectal cancers are microsatellite unstable due to methylation of the *MLH1* gene promoter during tumourigenesis. Methylation-sensitive primers may be used in PCR reactions to demonstrate that this is the cause of loss of expression of the *MLH1* gene and microsatellite instability in these tumours [6]. Alternatively, these tumours characteristically have mutations of *BRAF* that are not seen in Lynch syndrome tumours [18].

Genetic testing

Genetic testing of DNA mismatch repair genes may be undertaken in families or individuals with suspected Lynch syndrome in whom microsatellite instability or loss of expression of a mismatch repair gene has been demonstrated in their tumour. The appropriate gene to investigate may be indicated by the loss of expression on immunohistochemistry.

Each Lynch syndrome family has a particular germline mutation of a DNA mismatch repair gene. In families in which a causative mutation has been identified, at-risk members may undergo predictive genetic testing to see if they have inherited the abnormality. This process involves genetic counselling prior to undertaking a genetic test. At-risk individuals are at a 1:2 risk of carrying the mutation.

In a proportion of Lynch syndrome families with microsatellite unstable cancers and loss of expression of a mismatch repair gene, it may not be possible to find germline alterations using current technology. These families still require on-going surveillance, with each at-risk individual being treated as though they had Lynch syndrome, as it cannot be excluded in any of them in the absence of an identified mutation.

Clinical management

Individuals with, or at risk of, Lynch syndrome should undergo regular surveillance to reduce their risk of developing or dying from Lynch syndrome-associated cancers.

Surveillance

Surveillance for colorectal cancer
There are prospective data to show that colonoscopic surveillance in Lynch syndrome leads to the detection of colorectal cancer at an earlier stage than in historical controls. There is one prospective controlled trial showing that surveillance led to a 43% reduction in the incidence of colorectal cancer [19]. Other studies have demonstrated a reduction in mortality associated with colonoscopic surveillance [20]. The use of narrow band imaging during colonoscopy has been demonstrated to increase the detection of small adenomas in Lynch syndrome patients [21].

The risk of developing colorectal cancer before the age of 25 is very low. It is recommended that colonoscopic surveillance should be undertaken every one to two years from the age of 20 or 25 with the upper age limit of surveillance depending on the patient's general state of health. The frequency of surveillance is greater than that for other familial colorectal cancers as the adenoma-carcinoma sequence appears to be accelerated in Lynch syndrome.

Surveillance for endometrial and ovarian cancer
As yet there are no prospective studies indicating that surveillance for endometrial cancer is beneficial. However, surveillance by gynaecological examination, transvaginal ultrasound and aspiration cytology starting from the age of 30-35 years may lead to the detection of premalignant lesions and early cancers. Prophylactic hysterectomy and salpingo-oophorectomy may be an option for women with Lynch syndrome after completion of their families [22].

Surveillance for other cancers

The lifetime risk of developing stomach, ureter, renal pelvis, small bowel, bile duct or brain tumours is less than 10%. The risk of developing gastric cancers may be higher in some countries. Surveillance for gastric cancer has been recommended if there is more than one case in the family with gastroduodenoscopy every 1-2 years from the age of 30-35. There is no prospective evidence of a benefit for surveillance for renal tract tumours but in families with more than one case abdominal ultrasound and urinary cytology may be undertaken every 1-2 years from the age of 30-35.

Familial colorectal cancer

In 50% of families fulfilling the Amsterdam criteria there is no evidence of microsatellite instability in the tumour or of a DNA mismatch repair gene defect. Prospective colonoscopic studies indicate that members of such families are at increased risk of developing colorectal neoplasia, although they do not appear to develop interval cancers during colonoscopic surveillance as has been seen in Lynch syndrome [23]. It is recommended that they should undergo colonoscopy every five years from the age of 25, with more frequent colonoscopies if adenomas are detected.

Treatment of colorectal cancer in Lynch syndrome

There is a debate as to whether individuals with Lynch syndrome who develop colorectal cancer should undergo a segmental or a subtotal colectomy. They are at increased risk of developing metachronous cancers, but this has to be weighed against the less good functional outcome from a subtotal colectomy. The options should be discussed with each patient.

As discussed in an earlier section, there is evidence that microsatellite unstable cancers do not respond to 5FU-based chemotherapy. There is limited evidence of a response to irinotecan [24]. Adjuvant or palliative chemotherapy needs to be discussed carefully with patients on the basis of up-to-date studies.

The future

A large number of individuals and families with Lynch syndrome remain unrecognised and undiagnosed. The evidence that microsatellite unstable tumours have a different response to chemotherapy should lead to a greater proportion of colorectal cancers undergoing testing and increased identification of Lynch syndrome families.

Developments such as narrow band imaging should increase the accuracy of colonoscopic surveillance, and dietary or pharmacological interventions in the future may reduce the incidence of cancer in gene carriers.

Chemoprevention holds some promise. A large randomised study, CAPP2 (Colorectal Adenoma/carcinoma Prevention Programme), of the effect of resistant starch and aspirin on the development of colorectal cancer in Lynch syndrome has been undertaken and is about to be published. A new trial, POET (Prevention Of Endometrial Tumours), has been initiated to investigate the role of progesterone-releasing intra-uterine devices in reducing the incidence of endometrial cancer.

Key points

- Lynch syndrome is an autosomal dominantly inherited syndrome characterised by the development of colorectal, endometrial and various other cancers.
- Lynch syndrome is caused by a mutation in one of the mismatch repair genes: *MLH1, MSH2, MSH6* or *PMS2*.
- Predictive genetic testing is available in Lynch syndrome families in whom the genetic defect has been identified.
- There is prospective evidence that colonoscopic surveillance reduces the incidence of and mortality from colorectal cancer.
- As yet there is no prospective evidence that surveillance for endometrial, gastric and renal tract cancers reduces mortality.
- Regional genetic clinics with registries are essential to ensure that at-risk family members undergo regular surveillance and are offered appropriate genetic counselling.

References

1. Warthin AS. Heredity with reference to carcinoma. *Arch Intern Med* 1913; 12: 546-55.
2. Lynch HT, Shaw MW, Magnuson CW, *et al.* Hereditary factors in cancer. Study of two large midwestern kindreds. *Arch Intern Med* 1966; 117: 206-12.
3. Bronner CE, Baker SM, Morrison PT, *et al.* Mutation in the DNA mismatch repair gene homologue *hMLH1* is associated with hereditary non-polyposis colon cancer. *Nature* 1994; 368: 258-61.
4. Fishel R, Lescoe MK, Rao MR, *et al.* The human mutator gene homolog *MSH2* and its association with hereditary nonpolyposis colon cancer. *Cell* 1993; 75: 1027-38.
5. Miyaki M, Konishi M, Tanaka K, *et al.* Germline mutation of *MSH6* as the cause of hereditary nonpolyposis colorectal cancer. *Nature Genet* 1997; 17: 271-2.
6. Nicolaides NC, Papadopoulos N, Liu B, *et al.* Mutations of two PMS homologues in hereditary nonpolyposis colon cancer. *Nature* 1994; 371: 75-80.
7. Nystrom-Lahti M, Kristo P, Nicolaides NC, *et al.* Founding mutations and Alu-mediated recombination in hereditary colon cancer. *Nature Med* 1995; 1: 1203-6.
8. Kane MF, Loda M, Gaida GM, *et al.* Methylation of the *hMLH1* promoter correlates with lack of expression of *hMLH1* in sporadic colon tumors and mismatch repair-defective human tumor cell lines. *Cancer Res* 1997; 57: 808-11.
9. Hampel H, Stephens JA, Pukkala E, *et al.* Cancer risk in hereditary nonpolyposis colorectal cancer syndrome: later age of onset. *Gastroenterology* 2005; 129: 415-21.
10. Vasen HFA, Moslein G, Alonso A, *et al.* Guidelines for the management of Lynch syndrome (hereditary nonpolyposis colorectal cancer). *J Med Genet* 2007; 44: 353-62.
11. Jass JR, Smyrk TC, Stewart SM, *et al.* Pathology of hereditary non-polyposis colorectal cancer. *Anticancer Research* 1994; 14: 1631-4.
12. Carethers JM, Chauhan DP, Fink D, *et al.* Mismatch repair proficiency and *in vitro* response to 5-fluorouracil. *Gastroenterology* 1999; 117: 123-31.
13. Jover R, Zapater P, Castells A, *et al.* Mismatch repair status in the prediction of benefit from adjuvant fluorouracil chemotherapy in colorectal cancer. *Gut* 2006; 55: 848-55.
14. Ribic CM, Sargent DJ, Moore MJ, *et al.* Tumor microsatellite-instability status as a predictor of benefit from fluorouracil-based adjuvant chemotherapy for colon cancer. *N Engl J Med* 2003; 349: 247-57.
15. Vasen HF, Watson P, Mecklin JP, Lynch HT. New clinical criteria for hereditary nonpolyposis colorectal cancer (HNPCC, Lynch syndrome) proposed by the International Collaborative group on HNPCC. *Gastroenterology* 1999; 116: 1453-6.
16. Hampel H, Frankel WL, Martin E, *et al.* Screening for the Lynch syndrome (hereditary nonpolyposis colorectal cancer). *N Engl J Med* 2005; 352: 1851-60.
17. Umar A, Boland CR, Terdiman JP, *et al.* Revised Bethesda guidelines for hereditary nonpolyposis colorectal cancer (Lynch syndrome) and microsatellite instability. *J Natl Cancer Inst* 2004; 96: 261-8.
18. Domingo E, Laiho P, Ollikainen M, *et al.* BRAF screening as a low-cost effective strategy for simplifying HNPCC genetic testing. *J Med Genet* 2004; 41: 664-8.
19. Dove-Edwin I, Sasieni P, Adams J, Thomas HJ. Prevention of colorectal cancer by colonoscopic surveillance in individuals with a family history of colorectal cancer: 16-year, prospective, follow-up study. *BMJ* 2005; 331: 1047.

20. Jarvinen HJ, Aarnio M, Mustonen H, *et al*. Controlled 15-year trial on screening for colorectal cancer in families with hereditary nonpolyposis colorectal cancer. *Gastroenterology* 2000; 118: 829-34.

21. East JE, Suzuki N, Stavrinidis M, *et al*. Narrow band imaging for colonoscopic surveillance in hereditary non-polyposis colorectal cancer. *Gut* 2008; 57: 65-70.

22. Schmeler KM, Lynch HT, Chen LM, *et al*. Prophylactic surgery to reduce the risk of gynecologic cancers in the Lynch syndrome. *N Engl J Med* 2006; 354: 261-9.

23. Dove-Edwin I, de Jong AE, Adams J, *et al*. Prospective results of surveillance colonoscopy in dominant familial colorectal cancer with and without Lynch syndrome. *Gastroenterology* 2006, 130: 1995-2000.

24. Fallik D, Borrini F, Boige V, *et al*. Microsatellite instability is a predictive factor of the tumor response to irinotecan in patients with advanced colorectal cancer. *Cancer Res* 2003; 63: 5738-44.

Chapter 7

Breast cancer

Fiona Lalloo MD FRCP
Consultant in Clinical Genetics
St Mary's Hospital, Manchester, UK

Background

Breast cancer is the most common form of cancer affecting women. One in nine to twelve women will develop the disease in their lifetime in the developed world. Every year 39,000 women develop the disease in England and Wales (population 55 million) and as a result, 13,000 will die (Cancer Research Campaign Statistics).

There are a number of risk factors that increase the risk of breast cancer including young age at menarche (<10 years), older age at delivery of first child, or nulliparity and older age at menopause. However, the strongest risk factor is that of family history. The risk to an individual increases with the increasing number of relatives affected with breast cancer and the decreasing age at which they are diagnosed.

Approximately 5-10% of breast cancer is genetic with a small proportion being due to high penetrance genes transmitted in an autosomal dominant fashion. A further proportion is due to a larger number of moderate penetrance genes and it is likely that further cases are due to lower penetrance genes that may be interacting to increase the risk of breast cancer.

There are a number of family history clinics for the assessment of an individual's risk of breast cancer nationally, with the aim of providing a network of services from primary, through secondary and into tertiary care. The referral pathways depend upon the level of assessed risk according to the NICE guidelines for familial breast cancer [1].

Genetics and clinical picture

High penetrance genes

In the last 15 years advances in the genetics of breast cancer have resulted in the cloning of *BRCA1* and *BRCA2*, pathogenic mutations which are known to increase the risk of breast cancer by 10-20-fold. Mutations in *TP53* also give a high risk of breast cancer although the frequency of germline mutations in this gene is much lower.

BRCA1

About 1 in 1,000 individuals carry a pathogenic mutation in *BRCA1* which accounts for about 10% of familial breast cancer.

Pathogenic mutations in *BRCA1* confer a lifetime risk of breast cancer between 80-85%, with increased relative risks at younger ages. For example, the relative risk of breast cancer between the ages of 30-39 is 33, but it drops to 14 between the ages of 60-69 years [2].

Pathogenic mutations also increase the lifetime risk of ovarian cancer, although this is not as age-dependent. Women may also have an increased risk of pancreatic malignancy. Men with mutations in *BRCA1* have a relative risk of cancer of 0.95 [3].

BRCA1 is a large gene with 24 exons, the largest being exon 11. Mutations are found throughout the gene, with the majority being frameshift mutations. Missense mutations only account for about 2% of mutations in *BRCA1* but may be difficult to interpret or distinguish from polymorphisms. Between 15-30% of mutations may be due to large rearrangements, including large deletions (whole exon) and insertions/duplications. There does not appear to be any genotype-phenotype correlation.

Although hundreds of unique pathogenic mutations have been described in *BRCA1*, within certain populations particular mutations are more common (founder mutations). For example, within the Ashkenazi Jewish population, two mutations, c.68_69delAG and c.5266dupC (previous nomenclature 185delAG and 5382insC) occur in about 1.2% of the population. The 5382insC mutation is also found in other eastern European populations. This facilitates mutation screening within these populations.

The major role of the BRCA1 protein appears to be DNA repair, including homologous recombination and nucleotide excision repair. However, it also has a function in the regulation of cell cycle progression, in particular, checkpoint control.

Clinical features of BRCA1

Breast cancers in women with *BRCA1* mutations often exhibit different pathology to those of *BRCA2* mutation carriers and non-inherited breast cancers. These cancers have been noted to have an increased frequency of pushing margins, a high degree of nuclear pleomorphism and high mitotic frequency, features suggestive of medullary carcinoma. Indeed, atypical medullary breast cancers have been observed more frequently with *BRCA1* mutations: 13% vs 3% in sporadic breast cancers. Breast malignancies in *BRCA1* mutation carriers are also more likely to be steroid receptor and Her-negative than sporadic cancers. Ductal carcinoma *in situ* (DCIS) is noted less frequently in *BRCA1* mutation carriers. It has recently been noted [4] that *BRCA1* cancers have a similar immunohistological profile to sporadic basal cell carcinomas (carcinomas expressing molecules normally seen in the basal/myoepithelial cells of the normal breast).

The prognosis of *BRCA1*-associated breast cancers has been reported as both better and worse than sporadic tumours, although the association with ER-negative tumours and basal carcinomas would support the hypothesis of worse prognosis.

Women with a pathological mutation in *BRCA1* have an increased risk of developing contralateral tumours of up to 60% (compared with 20% in sporadic cancers).

The ovarian tumours associated with *BRCA1* mutations are usually serous epithelial carcinomas. Endometrioid and clear-cell carcinomas have been reported but mucinous and borderline tumours are not seen with *BRCA1* mutations [5]. Primary peritoneal malignancies have been described in *BRCA1* mutation carriers.

BRCA2

BRCA2 mutations account for about 10% of families with breast and ovarian cancer. Mutations in this gene confer a breast cancer lifetime risk of around 80%. However, one particular mutation in the Ashkenazi Jewish population, c.5946delT (6174 delT), has a much lower penetrance with some studies suggesting a lifetime risk of breast cancer of about 30%. The ovarian risk associated with pathogenic mutations is up to 20%. There is more variability of risks associated with mutations in *BRCA2* which suggests that this is a modifiable gene. The relative risks of cholangiocarcinoma, pancreatic and gastric cancers are also increased. Families are often seen with a wide variety of malignancies at a younger age than in the general population.

Male carriers of *BRCA2* mutations have an increased risk of prostate cancer with a lifetime risk of 14%.

As with *BRCA1*, *BRCA2* is a large gene with 27 exons encoding a 3418 amino acid protein, with exon 11 being the largest. Mutations occur throughout the gene, again the majority being frameshifts. There are a large number of missense mutations found within *BRCA2*, but the pathogenicity of these may be difficult to establish. Large gene rearrangements have also been described in *BRCA2* mutations. There is an area within exon 11 called the ovarian cluster region (OCR) flanked by nucleotides 3035 and 6629. Within the OCR there is a higher risk of ovarian cancer, about 20% as compared with mutations outside this region conferring a risk of about 10% [6].

BRCA2 is known to be involved in DNA repair. It facilitates homologous recombination and is involved with double strand break repair. It interacts directly with RAD51 forming a complex and holding it in an inactive state. Cells that lack BRCA1 or BRCA2 are hypersensitive to DNA-damaging agents with resulting double-stranded breaks. These are then repaired by an error prone mechanism such as non-homologous end joining, resulting in chromosomal rearrangements and instability. This chromosomal instability is a crucial feature of carcinogenesis.

Biallelic mutations in *BRCA2* have been shown to cause Fanconi anaemia, a condition causing developmental anomalies including short stature, microcephaly and radial ray abnormalities as well as predisposing to childhood solid tumours and haematological malignancies.

Clinical features of BRCA2
Breast cancer pathology is not as clearly defined with *BRCA2* mutations as *BRCA1*. The tumours appear to have less tubule differentiation and both increased and decreased mitotic rates compared with sporadic tumours have been reported. Lobular carcinoma has been reported more commonly with *BRCA2*-associated tumours whereas they are very uncommon with *BRCA1*-associated tumours. DCIS is more common in *BRCA2* tumours.

These tumours are more frequently ER-positive than control tumours although of higher grade. Overall, *BRCA2* tumours tend to have similar features to sporadic breast cancers unlike *BRCA1* tumours.

The prognosis of these tumours is the same as population breast cancers.

Ovarian carcinomas associated with *BRCA2* have similar features of those associated with *BRCA1*. Borderline and mucinous tumours are not part of the clinical picture. The prognosis of *BRCA2*-associated ovarian cancers is better than the general population, probably due to a better response to platinum-based therapies.

TP53
Somatic mutations in the *TP53* gene are common in solid tumours. Inherited germline mutations are rare but are known to result in Li-Fraumeni syndrome (LFS). LFS causes childhood tumours (typically soft tissue and osteosarcomas, gliomas or adrenocortical carcinomas) and very early onset breast cancer (50% of female gene carriers have developed breast cancer by 30 years of age). Over 70% of classical LFS

families have inherited *TP53* mutations [7]. There is good *in vitro* evidence to suggest patients with LFS have an abnormal response to low-dose radiation with defective apoptosis [8]. Recognition of this syndrome is important as these women should avoid radiotherapy if possible due to an increased risk of second primary malignancies.

Li-Fraumeni syndrome only accounts for about 1% of breast cancers but mutations in *TP53* confer an 18-fold increased risk of breast cancer before the age of 45 years compared with the general population.

TP53 was first identified in 1979 and now is known to be the most frequently altered gene in human tumours. Somatic mutations occur throughout the gene although there is clustering of mutations within the central part. Germline mutations have also been described throughout the gene. *TP53* consists of 11 exons, with the core DNA binding domain being encoded by exons 4-8. *TP53* is essential in cell cycle control, resulting in either a delay in cell cycle progression or apoptosis.

Moderate penetrance genes

There are four genes in which mutations result in a relative risk of breast cancer of 2-4 fold. These are rare genes with a population frequency of less than 0.6%. Whilst *BRCA1* and *BRCA2* mutations may account for up to 20% of familial breast cancer, these genes together account for only about 2.5%. The phenotypes associated with these mutations have not been clearly delineated and, therefore, the clinical utility of these genotypes has yet to be established.

ATM

Ataxia telangiectasia is an autosomal recessive condition due to homozygous mutations in *ATM*. Clinically this condition results in progressive cerebellar ataxia and oculomotor apraxia, conjunctival telangiectasia, immunodeficiency and an increased risk of malignancy including breast cancer.

It has been suggested for a number of years that heterozygotes of *ATM* have an increased risk of breast cancer [9], although this has been very controversial. However, recent studies [10] have confirmed an increased relative risk of breast cancer of 2.23 (95% CI 1.16-4.28) in heterozygotes of *ATM*. This relative risk increases under the age of 50 years.

Mutations described in *ATM* include truncating mutations, mutations affecting splice sites and missense mutations.

ATM protein is involved in the response to double stranded DNA breaks in a pathway that includes P53, BRCA1 and CHEK2.

It is difficult to assess the clinical utility of genetic testing for ATM mutations at present. The penetrance of the gene is about 15% and estimating which mutation carriers will develop breast cancer is not possible. However, these women may merit different approaches to treatment of breast cancer due to the increased radiosensitivity associated with mutations in *ATM*.

CHEK2

The checkpoint kinase gene, *CHEK2*, encodes a protein that is a signalling component in the cellular response to DNA damage. It is involved in the same pathway as P53 and BRCA1. *CHEK2* is a tumour suppressor gene and somatic mutations have been identified in a number of malignancies. A particular germline mutation, 1100delC, has been shown to give a relative risk of breast cancer of 2.34 (95% CI 1.72-3.2) [11]. It is thought to be present in 1% of the population and 4.2% of breast cancer families, although the frequency of the mutation varies between populations. A number of other rare mutations of *CHEK2* have been reported in breast cancer families but the clinical significance of these is unclear.

Carriers of the 1100delC mutation have an increased risk of bilateral breast cancer. Originally it was suggested that it may also contribute to male breast cancer but this has not been verified. There does not appear to be an increased risk of other malignancies with *CHEK2* mutations.

As with *ATM*, the clinical management of these women is unclear.

BRIP1

BRIP1 encodes for a protein that was identified as a binding partner of BRCA1 and was therefore investigated as a breast cancer predisposing gene. In 2006 truncating mutations were identified in breast cancer families [7]. Segregation analysis identified a relative risk of breast cancer of 2.0 (95% CI 1.2-3.2).

Biallelic mutations of *BRIP1* cause Fanconi anaemia complementation group J. Whilst biallelic mutations in *BRCA2* also cause Fanconi anaemia, there are differences in the phenotypes with a much lower rate of childhood solid tumours in FANC-J.

PALB2

PALB2 (partner and localizer of *BRCA2*) encodes for a protein that interacts with BRCA2 during homologous recombination and double strand break repair.

Mutations in this gene were identified in breast cancer families negative for mutations in *BRCA1/2*. The relative risk of breast cancer associated with mutations in *PALB2* is estimated at 2.3 (95% CI 1.4-3.9). It has been suggested that there is a Finnish founder mutation in this gene resulting in a slightly higher relative risk of breast cancer within this population.

Biallelic mutations in *PALB2* have been shown to cause Fanconi anaemia complementation group N. This type of Fanconi anaemia is similar to that caused by biallelic mutations in *BRCA2* (FANC-D1).

Low penetrance genes

It has been suggested that a number of common alleles will give a slightly increased risk of breast cancer and that some of these alleles may have a cumulative effect. They may in fact act as modifiers of *BRCA1/2*.

There is now evidence for a number of low-risk breast cancer predisposition alleles [8] (see Table 1), although as with the moderate risk alleles, this information is not yet being used in a clinical context.

Table 1. Low penetrance breast cancer variants.

Gene	Locus	SNP	Heterozygote OR (95% CI)	Homozygote OR (95% CI)
FGFR2	10q26	rs2981582	1.23 (1.18-1.28)	1.63 (1.53-1.72)
TNRC9	16q12	rs3803662	1.23 (1.18-1.29)	1.39 (1.26-1.45)
MRPS30	2q35	rs10941679	1.11 (1.03-1.20)	1.44 (1.30-1.58)
MAP3K1	5q11	rs889312	1.13 (1.09-1.18)	1.27 (1.19-1.36)
CASP8	2q33	rs1045485	0.89 (0.85-0.94)	0.74 (0.62-0.87)
LSP1	11p15	rs3817198	1.06 (1.02-1.11)	1.17 (1.08-1.25)

Diagnosis

Referral criteria

In 2004, the National Institute for Health and Clinical Excellence (NICE) published guidelines for referral and management of familial breast cancer [1], which were subsequently updated in 2006. These guidelines manage the referral pathway for women from primary to secondary through to tertiary care. The aim of the guidelines is for women to be stratified according to average, moderate and high risk of breast cancer, with only those at high risk with a high probability of mutations in BRCA1/2 being referred to the regional genetic services. Women at moderate risk should be assessed and managed in secondary care, ideally in association with breast units.

Risk assessment

Broadly speaking a woman's risk of breast cancer increases with the increasing number of relatives with associated cancers and the decreasing age at which those relatives were diagnosed.

Important factors within the family history include:

- Young age at onset of the disease.
- Bilateral disease.
- Multiple cases on one side of the family.

The most important tool for risk assessment is an accurate three-generation pedigree. A paternal history is as important as a maternal history especially considering that men are more likely to be non-penetrant gene carriers. The number of unaffected family members should be considered as large numbers may decrease the likelihood of a history being genetic.

There are a few families where it is possible to be sure of dominant inheritance (Figure 1). This makes risk assessment straightforward as it depends on the prior probability of inheriting the mutation and the penetrance of the gene. However, in the absence of a dominant family history, risk estimation is based on large epidemiological studies. These demonstrate a 1.5-3-fold increased risk with a family history of a single affected relative.

There are different ways of utilising these models, either using them manually to estimate risk or using computer programs that utilise epidemiological data. Some of the computer programmes also include the likelihood of detecting a *BRCA1/2* mutation within a given pedigree.

The models in wide use for risk estimation include the Claus model [12], Gail model [13], BRCAPRO and the Tyrer-Cuzick model. The Claus model is used mainly in the UK for manual risk estimation, whereas the other three are computerised.

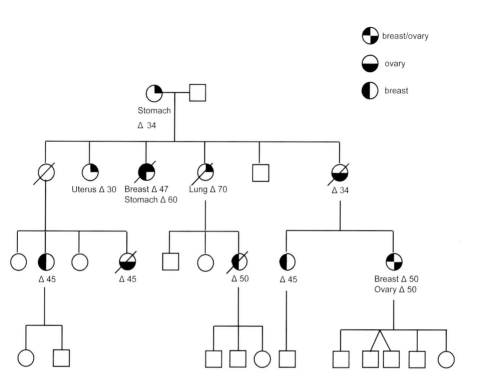

Figure 1. Clearly autosomal dominant history of breast and ovarian cancer. (∆=age at diagnosis).

Amir *et al* [14] assessed the accuracy of the different risk estimation models using data from 1,933 women with a family history of breast cancer in a screening programme. Fifty-two of these women developed a malignancy which was detected during the screening programme. All models were applied to this group of women and the Tyrer-Cuzick model was the most consistently accurate in predicting breast cancer risk. The other models significantly underestimated the risks. However, the Claus model can be modified by altering the risks according to hormonal factors (using the manual model of risk estimation).

Genetic testing

High-risk families should be referred to a regional genetics department to discuss the likelihood of developing a genetic test within a family. Predictive genetic testing (testing of unaffected at-risk individuals) is only possible if a mutation has been identified within a family, usually using a sample of DNA from a person with a malignancy. If a sample cannot be obtained from a living affected individual, in most cases genetic screening will not be undertaken. The exception to this is if the family is from a population with specific founder mutations such as the Ashkenazi population.

The NICE guidelines state that mutation screening should be offered in families if there is a greater than 20% probability of detecting a *BRCA1/2* mutation. There are a number of methods of determining the likelihood of detecting a *BRCA1/2* mutation within a given family. These include computer models: BOADICEA, BRCAPRO, and Tyrer-Cuzick. The computer models require inputting of data to the computer and may take around 5-10 minutes per family. Figure 2 shows a risk assessment and probability of *BRCA* mutation from the Tyrer-Cuzick programme. Myriad provides prevalence tables using family histories and data obtained from their clinical testing service. The Manchester scoring system is a tabulated scoring system that can be used easily in 1-2 minutes. A recent publication [15] validated these models using data from 2140 families. This study demonstrated that BOADICEA outperformed the other models. Both the BOADICEA and Manchester score incorporate information about pancreatic and prostate cancers into their systems unlike the other models. All these models could be improved by incorporating tumour pathology information.

Once a mutation is known within a family, predictive genetic testing becomes available. This then allows the identification of mutation carriers with the potential for targeted screening and intervention. Patients undergoing predictive testing are seen in the regional genetics service at least twice so that they are fully informed about the cancer risk associated with mutations and the implications to themselves and the wider family. Some individuals feel that psychologically they are unable to cope with the information that they are definitely at high risk of malignancy and therefore

Age of person is 32 years
Age at menarche is unknown
Age at first birth was 28 years
Person is premenopausal

Risk after 10 years is 1.736%
10-year population risk is 0.695%
Lifetime risk is 23.13%
Lifetime population risk is 10.16%
Probability of a *BRCA1* gene is 0.695%
Probability of a *BRCA2* gene is 0.448%

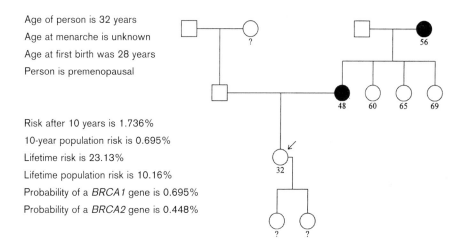

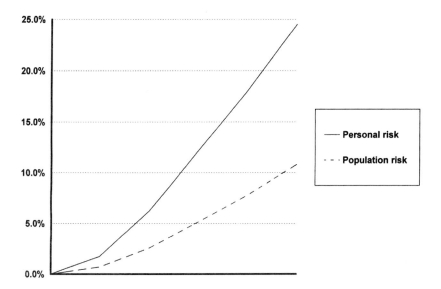

Figure 2. A risk assessment and probability of *BRCA* mutation from the Tyrer-Cuzick programme.

choose to not have a genetic test. They then avail themselves of the screening and surgical options.

Predictive genetic testing for *BRCA1/2* mutations is only offered to individuals over the age of consent.

Clinical management

The NICE guidelines clearly categorise the management of women at increased risk into:

◆ Moderate risk: a lifetime risk of one in six to one in four or a ten-year risk of 3-8% between 40-49 years.
◆ High risk: a lifetime risk of one in three or higher or a ten-year risk of greater than 8% between 40-49 years.

Moderate-risk women should be managed in secondary care and high-risk women in tertiary care.

Surveillance for breast cancer

Mammography

Currently, the National Health Service in the UK provides three-yearly mammography for women in the general population between the ages of 50 and 67 years (National Health Service Breast Screening Programme [NHSBSP]). Women with an increased risk of double the population risk or higher are eligible for screening on an annual basis from the age of 40.

If they are seen within an audited programme, screening can start from 35 years of age or five years under the youngest diagnosis of breast cancer within the family. Women whose lifetime risk of breast cancer is greater than one in four are also eligible for more frequent mammography as part of a research study or audited system. This often equates to 18-monthly mammograms between the ages of 50-60 years.

Magnetic resonance imaging (MRI)

There have been a number of trials assessing the utility of MRI screening for women at increased risk of breast cancer. In women with *BRCA1/2* mutations, mammography only detects about 50% of lesions due to a variety of factors including increased density of breast tissue in young women. MRI has greater sensitivity and specificity than mammography alone. However, MRI does have limited sensitivity in detecting DCIS, which may be an issue with *BRCA2* mutation carriers and, therefore, both MRI and mammography should be carried out.

The NICE guidelines state that MRI should be available for:

- Women aged 20-29 if they carry a *TP53* mutation.
- Women aged 30-39 if they:
  - carry a *TP53*, *BRCA1* or *BRCA2* mutation;
  - have a 50% risk of *TP53*, *BRCA1* mutation in either a family where a mutation has been identified or there is a greater than 60% chance of a mutation;
  - have a ten-year risk greater than 8%.
- Women aged 40-49 years if they:
  - carry a *TP53*, *BRCA1* or *BRCA2* mutation;
  - have a 50% risk of *TP53*, *BRCA1* mutation in either a family where a mutation has been identified or there is a greater than 60% chance of a mutation;
  - have a ten-year risk greater than 20%.

Currently, screening is on an *ad hoc* basis due to difficulties with funding, but the aim is that MRI and mammographic screening for women with an increased risk of breast cancer will be under the remit of the NHSBSP.

Surveillance for ovarian cancer

Women with *BRCA1/2* have a lifetime risk of ovarian cancer between 10-50%. The estimate of a given woman's risk depends upon the likelihood of a *BRCA1/2* mutation within the family. Currently this risk of ovarian cancer is managed by offering annual transvaginal ultrasound and

CA125 screening. However, there are concerns about the efficacy of screening [16] and all women eligible are therefore offered entry to UKFOCSS (UK familial ovarian cancer screening study)(www.pfsearch.ukcrn.org.uk). The aim of this study is to establish whether this form of screening works.

Prevention

Risk-reducing mastectomy

One of the options for women at high risk of breast cancer is to consider risk-reducing mastectomy as a prevention of breast cancer. There is good evidence to suggest that this will give a risk reduction of 90% [17, 18], although long-term follow-up of women with mutations undergoing surgery is not yet possible.

None of the different surgical procedures will completely remove all breast tissue, and there will therefore always be a small residual risk of breast malignancy. The prime aim of surgery is to remove breast tissue with cosmesis as a secondary aim. Both of these issues need to be discussed with individual women prior to surgery, along with issues surrounding general surgical and anaesthetic risks.

Whilst there have been few long-term studies on the psychological effects of surgery, most studies suggest significant benefit to women who choose this option compared with those that do not in terms of anxiety and cancer-related worry. It is important that protocols including psychological support are in place for any women considering surgery. The protocol in Manchester [19] includes two sessions with a clinical geneticist to discuss issues around genetic testing and risk, a session with a psychiatrist/psychologist to discuss body image and then sessions with the surgeons to discuss the different surgical options. The aim of the protocol is to ensure that patients are fully informed and as prepared as possible for surgery.

Risk-reducing oophorectomy

The management of choice for the ovarian risk in women with *BRCA1/2* mutations is risk-reducing oophorectomy once they have completed their family. Whilst UKFOCCS is still recruiting, early data [16] from regional genetic centres in the UK suggest that screening is not effective at detecting early stage ovarian cancer in mutation carriers. The tissues at risk include the ovaries and the fallopian tubes and therefore patients should be offered bilateral salpingo-oophorectomy (BSO). This reduces the risk of ovarian cancer by 90% as well as decreasing the risk of breast cancer if performed under 40-45 years of age [20].

Undergoing BSO at a young age will put women into menopause at an early age. The preliminary data regarding BSO in *BRCA1* mutation carriers suggest that the protection against breast cancer afforded by early surgery is unaffected by the type of HRT used. However, the Million Women study [21] suggests that the risk of breast cancer is lowest with oestrogen-only HRT which can only be used following hysterectomy. Therefore, any discussion of risk-reducing oophorectomy should include the risks and benefits of surgery, HRT and whether to include a hysterectomy.

Diet

Weight gain as an adult is clearly associated with an increased risk of postmenopausal breast cancer. This is also true for women with a family history of breast cancer. As such, there are a number of trials ongoing involving calorie restriction to determine whether this is a strategy for prevention of breast cancer within the family history group of patients.

Chemoprevention

Removing the effect of oestrogen from the breast has been shown to be useful as an adjunct to treating breast cancer and has therefore been suggested as a preventative measure.

Tamoxifen is known to reduce the risk of contralateral breast cancer in women with a previous breast primary. An American study [22] demonstrated a risk reduction of 40-50% in women with an increased lifetime risk who were given tamoxifen. However, smaller studies did not support this. Whilst the UK IBIS (International Breast Intervention Study [23]) demonstrated a 33% risk reduction with the use of tamoxifen (68 breast cancers *vs* 101), there are concerns over the increased risk of endometrial malignancy and thromboembolic events associated with the use of this drug. As such it has yet to be licensed in the UK for prevention of breast cancer, although it is licensed and used in the USA.

There are a number of ongoing studies assessing the use of aromatase inhibitors as chemopreventive agents.

The future

Targeted therapies

Given that *BRCA1* and *BRCA2* tumours seem to have different gene expression profiles from each other and sporadic tumours, it may be that they will respond differently to chemotherapeutic agents. Early *in vitro* studies have demonstrated that absence of BRCA2 protein results in increased sensitivity to paclitaxel, cisplatin and camptothecin. However, the studies regarding *BRCA1* are confused, with some cell lines suggesting increased sensitivity to paclitaxel and others suggesting increased resistance to this agent. There are no randomised controlled *in vivo* studies of treatment of *BRCA1/2* mutation carriers. Retrospective studies have demonstrated a differential response to neoadjuvant chemotherapy for breast cancers and an historical study suggests that the adverse prognosis in women with *BRCA1* mutations was only if they had not received chemotherapy.

Due to the controversy regarding response to platinum-based chemotherapy and taxanes, there is an ongoing Phase II study of carboplatin *vs* docetaxel for mutation carriers with metastatic breast cancer.

BRCA1 and BRCA2 are involved in homologous recombination as a double stranded DNA repair mechanism. PARP (Poly[ADP-ribose]polymerase) is involved in single stranded DNA repair. Inactivation of PARP results in spontaneous single stranded breaks being forced into double stranded DNA breaks. If BRCA1 and BRCA2 are inactive, these cells are not able to repair DNA damage and die. *In vivo* BRCA1/2-deficient cells are 2-3 times more sensitive to PARP inhibitors than wild-type cells. This may result in high therapeutic activity of this agent along with low toxicity.

There is currently an ongoing Phase II Proof of Principle Trial [24] of the activity of a PARP-1 inhibitor, in known carriers of a *BRCA1* or *BRCA2* mutation with locally advanced or metastatic breast or advanced ovarian cancer.

It is hoped that these agents will be effective, but this may depend on the rapid identification of mutation carriers at diagnosis of malignancy. Whilst techniques are being developed to look for 'signatures of BRCA-ness' in tumours, it is important that surgeons and oncologists enquire about family history. A three-generational pedigree is currently the most effective way of identifying individuals/families with a high probability of carrying a mutation.

Key points

◆ Familial breast cancer accounts for 5-10% of all breast cancer.

◆ *BRCA1* and *BRCA2* mutations account for about 20% of familial breast cancer. They are inherited in an autosomal dominant manner.

◆ A minority of patients with a family history are eligible for genetic testing.

◆ NICE has issued guidelines on the management of familial breast cancer.

◆ High-risk individuals should be seen in a tertiary regional genetics centre to discuss genetic testing, screening and preventative options.

◆ Clinical trials of targeted treatment for women with known mutations and breast or ovarian cancer are ongoing.

References

1. NICE and National Collaborating Centre for Primary Care. Clinical Guidelines and Evidence Review for The Classification and Care of Women at Risk of Familial Breast Cancer, 2004: http://www.nice.org.uk/CG041.

2. Antoniou A, Pharoah PD, Narod S, *et al.* Average risks of breast and ovarian cancer associated with *BRCA1* or *BRCA2* mutations detected in case series unselected for family history: a combined analysis of 22 studies. *Am J Hum Genet* 2003; 72: 1117-30.

3. Thompson D, Easton DF. Cancer incidence in *BRCA1* mutation carriers. *J Natl Cancer Inst* 2002; 94: 1358-65.

4. Lakhani SR, Reis-Filho JS, Fulford L, *et al.* Prediction of *BRCA1* status in patients with breast cancer using estrogen receptor and basal phenotype. *Clin Cancer Res* 2005; 11: 5175-80.

5. Evans DG, Young K, Bulman M, *et al.* Probability of *BRCA1/2* mutation varies with ovarian histology: results from screening 442 ovarian cancer families. *Clin Genet* 2008; 73: 338-45.

6. Gayther SA, Mangion J, Russell P, *et al.* Variation of risks of breast and ovarian cancer associated with different germline mutations of the *BRCA2* gene. *Nat Genet* 1997; 15: 103-5.

7. Seal S, Thompson D, Renwick A, *et al.* Truncating mutations in the Fanconi anemia J gene *BRIP1* are low-penetrance breast cancer susceptibility alleles. *Nat Genet* 2006; 38: 1239-41.

8. Easton DF, Pooley KA, Dunning AM, *et al.* Genome-wide association study identifies novel breast cancer susceptibility loci. *Nature* 2007; 447: 1087-93.

9. Swift ML, Reitnauer PJ, Morrell D, *et al.* Breast and other cancers in families with ataxia telangiectasia. *N Engl J Med* 1987; 316: 1289-94.

10. Thompson D, Duedal S, Kirner J, *et al.* Cancer risks and mortality in heterozygous *ATM* mutation carriers. *J Natl Cancer Inst* 2005; 97: 813-22.

11. CHEK2 Breast Cancer Case Control Consortium. *CHEK2**1100delC and susceptibility to breast cancer: a collaborative analysis involving 10,860 breast cancer cases and 9,065 controls from 10 studies. *Am J Hum Genet* 2004; 74: 1175-82.

12. Claus EB, Risch N, Thompson WD. Autosomal dominant inheritance of early-onset breast cancer; implications for risk prediction. *Cancer* 1994; 73: 643-51.

13. Speigelman D, Colditz GA, Hunter D, *et al.* Validation of the Gail *et al* model for predicting individual breast cancer risk. *J Natl Cancer Inst* 1994; 86: 600-7.

14. Amir E, Evans, DG, Shenton A, *et al.* Evaluation of breast cancer risk assessment packages in the family history evaluation and screening programme. *J Med Genet* 2003; 40: 807-14.

15. Antoniou A, Hardy R, Walker L, *et al.* Predicting the likelihood of carrying a *BRCA1* or *BRCA2* mutation: validation of BOADICEA, BRCAPRO, IBIS, Myriad and the Manchester scoring system using data from UK genetics clinics. *J Med Genet* 2008;

16. Stirling D, Evans DG, Pichert G, *et al.* Screening for familial ovarian cancer: failure of current protocols to detect ovarian cancer at an early stage according to the

International Federation of Gynecology and Obstetrics system. *J Clin Oncol* 2005; 23: 5588-96.

17. Hartmann LC, Schaid DJ, Woods JE, *et al*. Efficacy of bilateral prophylactic mastectomy in women with a family history of breast cancer. *N Engl J Med* 1999; 340: 77-84.

18. Meijers-Heijboer H, van Geel B, van Putten WL, *et al*. Breast cancer after prophylactic bilateral mastectomy in women with a *BRCA1* or *BRCA2* mutation. *N Engl J Med* 2001; 345: 159-64.

19. Lalloo F, Hopwood P, Baildam A, *et al*. Preventative mastectomy in women with an increased lifetime risk of breast cancer. *Eur J Surg Oncol* 2000; 26: 711-3.

20. van Roosmalen MS, Verhoef LC, Stalmeier PF. *et al*. Decision analysis of prophylactic surgery or screening for *BRCA1* mutation carriers: a more prominent role for oophorectomy. *J Clin Oncol* 2002; 20: 2092-100.

21. Beral V. Breast cancer and hormone-replacement therapy in the Million Women Study. *Lancet* 2003; 362: 419-27.

22. Fisher B, Costantino JP, Wickerham DL, *et al*. Tamoxifen for prevention of breast cancer: report of the National Surgical Adjuvant Breast and Bowel Project P-1 Study. *J Natl Cancer Inst* 1998; 90: 1371-88.

23. Cuzick J, Forbes J, Edwards R, *et al*. First results from the International Breast Cancer Intervention Study (IBIS-I): a randomised prevention trial. *Lancet* 2002; 360: 817-24.

24. National Cancer Research Network (NCRN). http://public.ukcrn.org.uk/Search/Study Detail.aspx?StudyID=4034.

Chapter 8

The gynaecologist and inherited cancer

Kathleen Schmeler MD
Assistant Professor of Gynecologic Oncology
The University of Texas M.D. Anderson Cancer Center
Houston, Texas, USA

Karen Lu MD
Professor of Gynecologic Oncology
The University of Texas M.D. Anderson Cancer Center
Houston, Texas, USA

Background

The gynaecologist and gynaecologic oncologist will likely encounter women in their practice who have a hereditary predisposition to ovarian and/or endometrial cancer. For both, asking patients about family history of cancer is a key component to identifying those at increased risk of having a hereditary cancer syndrome. The two main syndromes that involve gynaecologic malignancies are hereditary breast ovarian cancer syndrome (HBOC) and Lynch (LS)/hereditary non-polyposis colorectal cancer (HNPCC) syndrome. This chapter will describe how a physician identifies ovarian or endometrial cancer patients with HBOC or LS. In addition, this chapter will describe gynaecologic prevention and screening strategies for high-risk women.

Genetics

Ovarian cancer and hereditary breast ovarian cancer syndrome

Overall, approximately 10% of epithelial ovarian cancers are attributable to a germline *BRCA1* or *BRCA2* mutation. Prior to the identification of these two genes, clinicians had observed that certain women with ovarian cancer had a strong family history of ovarian and breast cancer suggestive of an autosomal dominant pattern of inheritance. The discovery of *BRCA1* and *BRCA2* in the early 1990s and the availability of genetic testing allows the precise genetic mutations of these genes to be identified in ovarian cancer patients with strong family histories of cancer. In addition, unaffected family members can undergo predictive genetic testing, thereby identifying women who are at extremely high risk of ovarian and breast cancer. A woman who carries a germline *BRCA1* mutation has a 20-40% lifetime risk of ovarian cancer. Germline *BRCA2* mutations are associated with a slightly lower 10-15% lifetime risk of ovarian cancer (Figure 1). These figures contrast with the 1.4% lifetime risk of ovarian cancer for women in the general population.

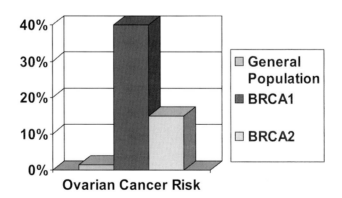

Figure 1. Lifetime risk of ovarian cancer in individuals with *BRCA1* and *BRCA2* mutations compared with the general population.

Endometrial cancer and Lynch syndrome

Lynch syndrome/hereditary non-polyposis colorectal cancer (HNPCC) is an autosomal dominant inherited cancer susceptibility syndrome caused by a germline mutation in one of the DNA mismatch repair genes (*MSH2*, *MLH1*, *MSH6*, *PMS2*). It is associated with early onset of cancer (age below 50 years) and the development of multiple cancer types, particularly colon and endometrial cancer.

The first description of a family with Lynch syndrome ('family G') was published in 1913 by Dr Alfred Warthin, a pathologist at the University of Michigan [1]. The initial proband was Dr Warthin's seamstress, who described an excessive number of family members with gastrointestinal and endometrial cancers, many at young ages. The seamstress eventually developed and died of endometrial cancer. In 1971, Dr Henry Lynch updated the original family G pedigree and further described the syndrome [2]. The specific molecular defect in family G was later identified as an *MSH2* mutation.

Clinical picture

Ovarian cancer and hereditary breast ovarian cancer syndrome

Women with *BRCA*-associated ovarian cancer are generally younger than women with sporadic ovarian cancer. *BRCA1* or *BRCA2*-associated ovarian cancers are predominantly high-grade papillary serous adenocarcinomas. Papillary serous carcinoma of the peritoneum (PSCP), or primary peritoneal cancer, is also part of the disease spectrum. In addition, primary fallopian tube cancers, which are serous adenocarcinomas, are also associated. Studies have demonstrated that women who have *BRCA*-associated ovarian cancers, as opposed to sporadic ovarian cancers, have improved survival [3]. It has been hypothesised that the improved survival is associated with an increased sensitivity of the ovarian tumour to chemotherapy.

Endometrial cancer and Lynch syndrome

In individuals with Lynch syndrome, the risk of colorectal cancer is approximately 80% for men and 40-60% for women, compared with a 4-5% risk in the general population (Figure 2). For women with Lynch syndrome, the risk of endometrial cancer is 40-60%, compared with a 3% risk in the general population. In addition, they have a 12% risk of ovarian cancer. Other cancer types associated with this syndrome include stomach (13% lifetime risk), small bowel (5% lifetime risk), renal pelvis and ureter (4% lifetime risk), brain (4% lifetime risk), and biliary tract (2% lifetime risk).

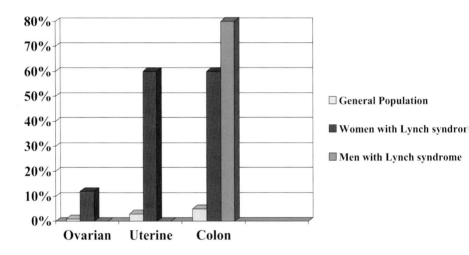

Figure 2. Lifetime risk of colon, endometrial and ovarian cancer in individuals with Lynch syndrome compared with the general population.

Diagnosis

Ovarian cancer and hereditary breast ovarian cancer syndrome

For a physician taking care of a woman with ovarian cancer, obtaining a personal and family history of cancer will assist in determining whether the patient may have a *BRCA* mutation. Prior personal history of breast cancer, family history of pre-menopausal breast cancer and ovarian cancer, as well as family history of male breast cancer can be red flags that suggest a *BRCA*-associated ovarian cancer. In addition, studies have shown that Ashkenazi Jewish women with ovarian cancer have a 40% chance of having one of three Ashkenazi Jewish founder mutations in *BRCA1* and *BRCA2* [4]. The Society of Gynecologic Oncologists (SGO) has set forth guidelines that identify women at strong risk for carrying a *BRCA* mutation [5]. Because genetic testing is most helpful when performed on a patient with cancer first, gynaecologists and gynaecologic oncologists who care for ovarian cancer patients should proactively identify those ovarian cancer patients who have a high likelihood of having a *BRCA* mutation.

Endometrial cancer and Lynch syndrome

Prior to the identification of the underlying genetic defects, the diagnosis of Lynch syndrome was based on clinical criteria. The initial criteria (Amsterdam I) were focused on colorectal cancer, and have been subsequently revised (Amsterdam II) to include all Lynch syndrome associated cancers (see pp90-91). The criteria include: i) three or more relatives with Lynch syndrome-associated cancers; ii) two affected relatives in successive generations; iii) one or more relatives with a Lynch syndrome- associated cancer diagnosed before the age of 50 years.

The underlying genetic defects causing Lynch syndrome are now known to be germline mutations in one of the DNA mismatch repair genes (*MLH1*, *MSH2*, *MSH6*, *PMS2*). Tumour studies, including immunohistochemistry and microsatellite instability testing, can be performed on paraffin-embedded tissue. These tumour studies allow clinicians an intermediate step prior to performing germline mutational analysis in evaluating individuals with Lynch syndrome-related malignancies. They can rule out Lynch syndrome in these patients, as well as simplify genetic testing by targeting particular genes in individuals with positive results.

In addition, the SGO recently published guidelines for referral of women at risk for Lynch syndrome [5]. The criteria include a combination of clinical and pathologic factors to help practitioners determine which patients should be referred for genetic risk assessment.

Clinical management

Ovarian cancer and hereditary breast ovarian cancer syndrome

Mutation carriers

With the availability of clinical genetic testing, more women with germline *BRCA1* or *BRCA2* mutations who are unaffected with cancer are presenting to their physicians for ovarian cancer screening and prevention. Unfortunately, there are currently no effective screening tests for the early detection of ovarian cancer. However, studies over the last decade have demonstrated that prophylactic bilateral salpingo-oophorectomy (BSO) is highly effective in decreasing the risk of ovarian cancer [6, 7]. During a consultation with a woman with a germline *BRCA* mutation regarding ovarian cancer risk management, the clinician needs to review all options for screening and prevention, and develop an acceptable, individualised strategy.

Surveillance for ovarian cancer

There are currently no effective screening tests for the early detection of ovarian cancer in high-risk women. However, given the substantial ovarian cancer risk in individuals with *BRCA1* and *BRCA2* mutations, consensus groups have recommended six-monthly screening with CA-125 and transvaginal ultrasound [8]. This recommendation is based on expert opinion only, and it is important for high-risk patients to understand the limitations of ovarian cancer screening.

CA-125

The measurement of serum CA-125 is clinically used in monitoring the disease status of women with ovarian cancer; however, it has limitations as a tool for early detection. While CA-125 is elevated in over 90% of stage III ovarian cancers, it is only elevated in approximately 50% of stage I ovarian cancers. In addition, using a cut-off value of 35U/ml, a number of non-malignant conditions including fibroids, endometriosis, menses, and pelvic inflammatory disease can cause elevated CA-125. There are currently ongoing studies that are examining the change over time of CA-125, rather than a single CA-125 level in order to improve the sensitivity and specificity of the marker. In addition, there are other new markers that are currently being testing either alone or in combination with CA-125.

Transvaginal ultrasound

Transvaginal ultrasound has been shown to increase sensitivity over CA-125 alone in identifying ovarian cancer, but has poor specificity. Retrospective studies that have examined the efficacy of transvaginal ultrasound with CA-125 in the early detection of ovarian cancer in high-risk populations have found that interval cancers occur despite screening and that screen-detected cancers are often at an advanced stage [9]. In the United Kingdom, a prospective study of annual transvaginal ultrasound with CA-125 every four months is ongoing for women at increased risk of ovarian cancer (United Kingdom Familial Ovarian Cancer Screening Study - UK FOCSS). The results of the prospective study will be important in further defining the efficacy of ovarian cancer screening.

Chemoprevention

Oral contraceptives are known to decrease ovarian cancer risk by 50% in the general population. Studies in *BRCA* mutation carriers show that this substantial decrease in risk of ovarian cancer is likely to hold true for women in this group [10]. In the general population, oral contraceptives are not believed to incur a higher risk of breast cancer. Studies have shown a slight increase in breast cancer risk with oral contraceptives in *BRCA* mutation carriers.

Risk-reducing surgery

Prophylactic BSO reduces the risk of developing ovarian cancer by approximately 85-95% [6, 7] In addition, performing the procedure premenopausally decreases the risk of breast cancer by at least 50%. Given the lack of an effective screening strategy and the lethality of ovarian cancer, women with germline *BRCA* mutations should be strongly counselled that prophylactic BSO is a reasonable and effective strategy to prevent ovarian cancer. However, the side effects of the procedure should also be discussed pre-operatively. For pre-menopausal women, the acute onset of menopausal symptoms including hot flashes and night sweats can have a significant adverse effect on quality of life. Long-term effects of the loss of endogenous oestrogen are on bone loss and atrophy of the vaginal epithelium. In women who have not had breast cancer, short-term hormone replacement therapy after prophylactic BSO is an option. A study by Rebbeck *et al* showed that hormone replacement therapy after BSO did not decrease the breast cancer benefit [11]. Long-term studies of side effects and quality of life are on-going by a number of groups and will be important for counselling women facing these choices.

Prophylactic BSO can be performed either laparoscopically or via laparotomy. In addition to thorough visualisation of the peritoneal surfaces in the abdomen and pelvis, a limited staging procedure, including washings and biopsies of suspicious areas should be performed. The ovaries should be removed in their entirety, and the fallopian tubes also need to be completely removed. The decision to remove the uterus should be made on an individual basis and based on other indications such as abnormal cervical smears in the past, history of tamoxifen use and other uterine abnormalities.

Studies by our group and others have shown that in the prophylactic BSO specimens, there is a defined risk of occult ovarian and fallopian tube cancers that are only found at the time of histopathologic review [12, 13]. The pathologist reviewing the case should completely examine the fallopian tubes and ovaries, which is not routinely performed. Serial sectioning should be performed at 2mm intervals and careful examination for occult tumours should occur. Finally, there remains a small risk of peritoneal cancer even after BSO. Patients should be counselled about the risk, but it is unclear whether any screening for peritoneal cancer is necessary. Overall, studies have shown that approximately 40-80% of women with *BRCA* mutations choose to undergo prophylactic BSO [14].

Endometrial cancer and Lynch syndrome

Surveillance for endometrial and ovarian cancer

Endometrial and ovarian cancer screening is not performed in the general population. For endometrial cancer, this is due to the low prevalence of disease, high survival rates and the occurrence of postmenopausal vaginal bleeding as an early symptom of disease. For ovarian cancer, screening is not performed in the general population due to the low prevalence of disease and lack of good screening modalities for diagnosis at an early stage.

Most women with Lynch syndrome-associated endometrial cancer present with stage I disease and have high overall survival rates, similar to women with sporadic endometrial cancer. It is unclear if endometrial cancer screening would improve morbidity and mortality in these high-risk patients. However, it is believed that surveillance could potentially decrease the amount of treatment needed by detecting the cancer at an earlier stage, when surgery alone is curative.

To date, suggested screening modalities include transvaginal ultrasound and endometrial biopsy. Two studies have examined the use of transvaginal ultrasound with the measurement of endometrial thickness as a screening modality for women with Lynch syndrome [15,16]. Both studies demonstrated limited efficacy, as well as high false-positive rates. This is likely due to the high variability in endometrial thickness in premenopausal women. A study by Lecuru and colleagues [17] evaluated 57 women with Lynch syndrome who underwent hysteroscopy with endometrial sampling as a screening modality for endometrial cancer. Two patients were diagnosed with endometrial cancer; however, both patients reported abnormal vaginal bleeding.

A recent Finnish study evaluated the combination of ultrasound and endometrial biopsy to screen for endometrial cancer in 175 women with Lynch syndrome [18]. There were no significant differences in ten-year survival rates between the women with endometrial cancer detected through screening (100%) and those detected due to symptoms (92%). However, 7% of the women in the surveillance group presented with stage III/IV disease, compared with 17% of the women who presented with symptoms. This study suggests that endometrial cancer screening in this high-risk cohort may have benefit in detecting disease at an earlier stage.

To date, there are no studies or data to support surveillance for ovarian cancer in women with Lynch syndrome. Despite limited information on the efficacy of surveillance in reducing endometrial and ovarian cancer risk in women with Lynch syndrome, the current gynaecologic cancer screening guidelines include annual endometrial sampling and transvaginal ultrasonography beginning at age 30 to 35 years [19]. Of note, these recommendations are based on expert opinion alone, as there have been no controlled studies demonstrating the efficacy of these screening modalities in young, premenopausal women with Lynch syndrome.

Chemoprevention

There are currently no studies specifically evaluating chemoprevention for gynaecologic malignancies in women with Lynch syndrome. However, in the general population, the Cancer and Steroid Hormone (CASH) case-control studies demonstrated a 50% reduction in the risk of endometrial and ovarian cancer with the use of oral contraceptive pills. In addition, progestin-containing agents have been shown to reverse or arrest disease progression in women with endometrial hyperplasia. In the absence of chemoprevention data specific to women with Lynch syndrome, the potential for cancer prevention with these agents can be extrapolated. However, further studies in this area are required as the gynaecologic cancers associated with Lynch syndrome may have important biologic differences from those in the general population. A multi-institutional study is currently underway comparing levonorgesterol oral contraceptive pills with depo-medroxyprogesterone acetate for chemoprevention in women with Lynch syndrome.

Risk-reducing surgery

Another option for women with Lynch syndrome is risk-reducing gynaecologic surgery. A recent retrospective cohort analysis by Schmeler and colleagues [20] evaluated 315 women with germline *MLH1*, *MSH2* or *MSH6* mutations. Patients who had undergone prophylactic hysterectomy with or without BSO, were compared with those who had not. No endometrial or ovarian cancers developed in those who had surgery, whereas 33% of those who did not have surgery developed endometrial cancer and 5.5% developed ovarian cancer. In this cohort, 100% of potential new endometrial and ovarian cancer cases were prevented with prophylactic surgery.

In this study, the median age at diagnosis was 46 years for endometrial cancer and 42 years for ovarian cancer. These findings were consistent with previous studies of women with Lynch syndrome that reported the mean age at endometrial cancer diagnosis to be 48 to 49 years, and the mean age at ovarian cancer diagnosis to be 42 years. Lindor *et al* [19] recently published updated recommendations for the care of individuals with an inherited predisposition to Lynch syndrome (Table 1). The authors performed a

Table 1. Recommended management for women with Lynch syndrome (adapted from Lindor *et al*, JAMA, 2006 [19]).

Intervention	Recommendation
History and physical exam	Every year beginning at age 21 with review of systems, education, and counselling regarding Lynch syndrome
Colonoscopy	Every 1-2 years beginning at age 20-25 years or 10 years younger than the youngest age at diagnosis in the family, whichever comes first. For *MSH6* families, begin at age 30.
Endometrial sampling	Every year beginning at age 30-35 years
Transvaginal ultrasound	Every year beginning at age 30-35 years
Urinalysis with cytology	Every 1-2 years beginning at age 25-35 years
Colorectal resection	Generally not recommended for primary prophylaxis, but if cancer diagnosed, subtotal colectomy is favoured
Hysterectomy with BSO	Discuss as option after childbearing complete

systematic review of the existing literature and recommended that prophylactic hysterectomy and BSO should be offered to all women aged 35 years or older who do not wish to preserve fertility. In addition, when a woman is undergoing surgery for colorectal cancer, consideration should be given to performing a concurrent prophylactic hysterectomy and BSO.

Previous studies of *BRCA* mutation carriers have reported that occult ovarian carcinomas can be diagnosed at the time of surgery. In the study by Schmeler et al [20], three women (5%) with Lynch syndrome who underwent prophylactic hysterectomy were found to have occult endometrial carcinomas. In addition, Chung and colleagues [21] published a case report about a woman with known Lynch syndrome who was found to have endometrial cancer with cervical involvement following a prophylactic hysterectomy. This patient required a second surgery for staging.

These findings emphasise the need for maintaining a high index of suspicion prior to and during prophylactic surgery in women with Lynch syndrome. Pre-operative assessment with endometrial biopsy, transvaginal ultrasound and CA125 levels should be considered. At the time of surgery, the uterus and ovaries should be carefully assessed. The pathologist should be advised of the high risk of endometrial and ovarian cancer, and the specimens carefully examined intra-operatively with frozen sections performed if indicated. In addition, the surgeon should be prepared to perform a complete staging operation in the case of occult carcinoma.

Previous studies in women with *BRCA* mutations have reported an incidence of primary peritoneal cancer following prophylactic BSO of 0.8-1.0% [6, 7]. To date, one case of primary peritoneal cancer following prophylactic BSO in a woman with Lynch syndrome has been reported. The patient underwent hysterectomy with BSO at age 44 and subsequently developed primary peritoneal cancer at the age of 56. Of note, she also developed a transitional cell carcinoma of the urethra at age 60 and two primary colon cancers at age 61. Longer follow-up and further study is necessary to better determine the risk of primary peritoneal cancer in women with Lynch syndrome following prophylactic BSO.

The disadvantages of prophylactic hysterectomy and BSO include surgical complications and premature menopause. The most common surgical complications associated with hysterectomy and BSO are bleeding, infection and injuries to the urinary tract and bowel. In premenopausal women, prophylactic BSO results in premature menopause. Symptoms may include hot flashes, vaginal dryness, sexual dysfunction and sleep disturbances. In addition, these women are at increased risk of osteoporosis. Many of these conditions can be managed with hormonal or non-hormonal medications. Unlike *BRCA* mutation carriers, there are no specific or unique contraindications to hormone replacement therapy in women with Lynch syndrome.

Synchronous and metachronous colorectal and endometrial or ovarian cancer

Women with Lynch syndrome are at high risk for developing synchronous or metachronous cancers [22, 23]. A woman with Lynch syndrome who survives colon cancer has a high likelihood of developing endometrial or ovarian cancer. Similarly, a woman who survives an endometrial or ovarian cancer is at high for developing colon cancer. Lu *et al* [23] reported on 117 women with Lynch syndrome with dual primary cancers. In 16 women (14%), the colorectal and gynaecologic cancers (endometrial or ovarian) were diagnosed simultaneously. Of the remaining 101 women, 52 (51%) had their endometrial or ovarian cancer diagnosed first and 49 women (49%) had their colon cancer diagnosed first.

In the study by Schmeler *et al* [20], 41 women (13%) were diagnosed with synchronous (three patients) or metachronous (38 patients) colorectal and endometrial or ovarian cancers. In 21 of these 41 women (51%), the gynaecologic cancer was diagnosed following treatment for colorectal cancer. The median time between the diagnoses of colon cancer and gynaecologic cancer was five years. The gynaecologic malignancies in these women could have been prevented if prophylactic hysterectomy and BSO had been performed at the time of their surgery for colorectal cancer. Strong consideration should be given to concurrent prophylactic hysterectomy and BSO in women undergoing surgery for colorectal cancer.

The future

The gynaecologist plays an important role in both the identification of women with hereditary cancer syndromes and in the management of high-risk women. Multidisciplinary efforts are crucial, given that women with both HBOC and Lynch syndrome may develop both gynaecologic and non-gynaecologic cancers and need to be extended. Further research is necessary to develop novel and effective screening and prevention strategies in women with these hereditary cancer syndromes.

Key points

- Approximately 10% of epithelial ovarian cancers are due to a *BRCA1* or *BRCA2* mutation.
- Risk of ovarian cancer with a *BRCA1* mutation is up to 46%, and with a *BRCA2* mutation up to 15%.
- BRCA-associated ovarian cancers are typically high-grade papillary serous adenocarcinomas. Primary fallopian tube and primary peritoneal cancers are also part of the disease spectrum.
- There is no proven efficacy for ovarian cancer screening in high-risk women.
- Prophylactic salpingo-oophorectomy decreases risk of ovarian cancer by more than 85-95%. The ovaries and fallopian tubes must be fully and carefully examined for microscopic cancer.
- Women with Lynch syndrome have a 40-60% lifetime risk of endometrial cancer.
- There is no proven efficacy for endometrial or ovarian cancer screening in women with Lynch syndrome.
- Prophylactic hysterectomy and salpingo-oophorectomy is a proven strategy for risk reduction in women with Lynch syndrome.
- Women with Lynch syndrome are at high risk of developing synchronous or metachronous gastrointestinal and gynaecologic cancers. In these women with dual primary cancers, approximately 50% will develop a gynaecologic cancer first.
- Most women with Lynch syndrome-associated endometrial cancer present with stage I disease and have high overall survival rates.

References

1. Warthin A. Heredity with reference to to carcinoma as shown by the study of the cases examined in the pathological library of the University of Michigan. *Arch of Intern Med* 1913; 12: 546-55.
2. Lynch HT, Krush AJ. Cancer family 'G' revisited: 1895-1970. *Cancer* 1971; 27: 1505-11.
3. Boyd J, Sonoda Y, Federici MG, *et al.* Clinicopathologic features of *BRCA*-linked and sporadic ovarian cancer. *JAMA* 2000; 283: 2260-5.
4. Moslehi R, Chu W, Karlan B, *et al. BRCA1* and *BRCA2* mutation analysis of 208 Ashkenazi Jewish women with ovarian cancer. *American Journal of Human Genetics* 2000; 66: 1259-72.
5. Lancaster JM, Powell CB, Kauff ND, *et al.* Society of Gynecologic Oncologists Education Committee statement on risk assessment for inherited gynecologic cancer predispositions. *Gynecologic Oncology* 2007; 107: 159-62.
6. Kauff ND, Satagopan JM, Robson ME, *et al.* Risk-reducing salpingo-oophorectomy in women with a *BRCA1* or *BRCA2* mutation. *N Engl J Med* 2002; 346: 1609-15.
7. Rebbeck TR, Lynch HT, Neuhausen SL, *et al.* Prophylactic oophorectomy in carriers of *BRCA1* or *BRCA2* mutations. *N Engl J Med* 2002; 346: 1616-22.
8. NCCN Clinical Practice Guidelines in Oncology: Genetic/Familial High-Risk Assessment: Breast and Ovarian. Rockledge, PA: National Comprehensive Cancer Network, 2006.
9. Gaarenstroom KN, van der Hiel B, Tollenaar RA, *et al.* Efficacy of screening women at high risk of hereditary ovarian cancer: results of an 11-year cohort study. *Int J Gynecol Cancer* 2006; 16 Suppl 1: 54-9.
10. Narod SA, Dube MP, Klijn J, *et al.* Oral contraceptives and the risk of breast cancer in *BRCA1* and *BRCA2* mutation carriers. *Journal of the National Cancer Institute* 2002; 94: 1773-9.
11. Rebbeck TR, Friebel T, Wagner T, *et al.* Effect of short-term hormone replacement therapy on breast cancer risk reduction after bilateral prophylactic oophorectomy in *BRCA1* and *BRCA2* mutation carriers: the PROSE Study Group. *J Clin Oncol* 2005; 23: 7804-10.
12. Lu KH, Garber JE, Cramer DW, *et al.* Occult ovarian tumors in women with *BRCA1* or *BRCA2* mutations undergoing prophylactic oophorectomy. *J Clin Oncol* 2000; 18: 2728-32.
13. Powell CB, Kenley E, Chen LM, *et al.* Risk-reducing salpingo-oophorectomy in *BRCA* mutation carriers: role of serial sectioning in the detection of occult malignancy. *J Clin Oncol* 2005; 23: 127-32.
14. Schmeler KM, Sun CC, Bodurka DC, *et al.* Prophylactic bilateral salpingo-oophorectomy compared with surveillance in women with *BRCA* mutations. *Obstet Gynecol* 2006; 108: 515-20.
15. Dove-Edwin I, Boks D, Goff S, *et al.* The outcome of endometrial carcinoma surveillance by ultrasound scan in women at risk of hereditary nonpolyposis colorectal carcinoma and familial colorectal carcinoma. *Cancer* 2002; 94: 1708-12.

16. Rijcken FE, Mourits MJ, Kleibeuker JH, *et al.* Gynecologic screening in hereditary nonpolyposis colorectal cancer. *Gynecologic Oncology* 2003; 91: 74-80.

17. Lecuru F, Metzger U, Scarabin C, *et al.* Hysteroscopic findings in women at risk of HNPCC. Results of a prospective observational study. *Fam Cancer* 2007; 6: 295-9.

18. Renkonen-Sinisalo L, Butzow R, Leminen A, *et al.* Surveillance for endometrial cancer in hereditary nonpolyposis colorectal cancer syndrome. *Int J Cancer* 2007; 120: 821-4.

19. Lindor NM, Petersen GM, Hadley DW, *et al.* Recommendations for the care of individuals with an inherited predisposition to Lynch syndrome: a systematic review. *JAMA* 2006, 296: 1507-17.

20. Schmeler KM, Lynch HT, Chen LM, *et al.* Prophylactic surgery to reduce the risk of gynecologic cancers in the Lynch syndrome. *N Engl J Med* 2006; 354: 261-9.

21. Chung L, Broaddus R, Crozier M, *et al.* Unexpected endometrial cancer at prophylactic hysterectomy in a woman with hereditary nonpolyposis colon cancer. *Obstet Gynecol* 2003; 102: 1152-5.

22. Mecklin JP, Jarvinen HJ. Clinical features of colorectal carcinoma in cancer family syndrome. *Dis Colon Rectum* 1986; 29: 160-4.

23. Lu KH, Dinh M, Kohlmann W, *et al.* Gynecologic cancer as a 'sentinel cancer' for women with hereditary nonpolyposis colorectal cancer syndrome. *Obstet Gynecol* 2005; 105: 569-74.

Chapter 9

Multiple endocrine neoplasia syndromes

Fausto Palazzo MS FRCS
Consultant Endocrine Surgeon
Hammersmith Hospital, London, UK
Honorary Senior Lecturer, Imperial College, London, UK

Karim Meeran MD FRCP
Professor of Endocrinology
Charing Cross and Hammersmith Hospitals, and
Imperial College, London, UK

Background

The first reports of combinations of endocrine pathologies occurring in the same patient date back to the beginning of the 20th century. In 1903, Jakob Erdheim reported the combination of an enlarged pituitary, a colloid goitre, three enlarged parathyroids and pancreatic necrosis in the autopsy of an acromegalic Viennese patient. A dozen or so other reports were reviewed in 1953 by Laurentius Underdahl who added the Mayo Clinic series of eight patients and coined the term multiple endocrine adenoma [1]. The following year Paul Wermer described a family with five affected members and proposed an autosomal dominant transmission [2].

Other endocrine combinations were also being noted, and in 1960 Alvin Hayles described a patient treated at the Mayo Clinic with bilateral phaeochromocytomas and a carcinoma of the thyroid with an amyloid stroma later confirmed to be a medullary thyroid cancer (MTC) [3]. The following year John Sipple of New York documented the eponymous syndrome when he described the autopsy of a 33-year-old male with bilateral phaeochromocytomas, MTC and parathyroid adenomas. He followed this with the finding of a disproportionately high prevalence of thyroid cancer in 537 patients with a phaeochromocytoma [4].

Wermer's and Sipple's syndromes became later known as multiple endocrine neoplasia (MEN) syndromes type 1 and 2, respectively, when Alton Steiner and colleagues added 168 New York patients to the existing literature and described the autosomal dominant inherited or sporadic combination of phaeochromocytoma, MTC and parathyroid tumours as MEN2. They named the syndrome characterised by diseases of the parathyroids, pituitary and pancreas, MEN1 [5]. It later became apparent that, whilst all MEN2 patients presented with phaeochromocytoma and MTC, there were two variants of the syndrome, since MEN2A patients had a normal appearance whereas MEN2B patients often manifested a marfanoid habitus, neuromas of the tongue and lips and an absence of parathyroid disease.

Genetics

MEN1

Multiple endocrine neoplasia type 1 syndrome is an autosomal dominant inherited disease with a high degree of penetrance. The gene responsible (*MEN1*) is found on the long arm of chromosome 11 (11q13) and encodes a 610 amino acid tumour suppressor protein called menin [6]. The protein is located primarily in the nucleus where it may bind to the transcription or DNA repair proteins [7]. Development of tumours in MEN1 syndrome conforms to Knudsen's two-hit hypothesis, where the carrier of a mutated, non-functioning allele (germline mutation) develops a tumour after inactivation of the other allele (somatic mutation) which opens the way for clonal proliferation.

Most *MEN1* mutations are associated with a decrease in menin which in turn is associated with an increase in damaged DNA, although the exact mechanism is unclear [8]. Whilst an error within the *MEN1* gene may lead to multiple endocrine pathologies it may also accompany sporadic single endocrine pathologies including parathyroid tumours, pancreatic neuroendocrine tumours, pituitary adenomas, lipomas and angiofibromas. Unlike MEN2 there is no genotype/phenotype correlation to justify gene sequencing for the purposes of the prediction of the severity of disease. Genetic testing identifies a mutation in up to 90% of index cases of MEN1.

MEN2

All three forms of MEN2 syndrome (2A, 2B and familial medullary thyroid cancer [FMTC]) are autosomal dominantly inherited and are caused by germline defects in the *RET* proto-oncogene found on chromosome 10, which are detectable in well over 90% of cases. The *RET* gene encodes a transmembrane tyrosine kinase receptor protein with downstream targets that remain incompletely understood. Apparently non-inherited somatic *RET* mutations are also involved in a significant number of papillary thyroid cancers (*RET-PTC* genes) and are associated with *RET* over-expression.

Given the tight genotype-phenotype correlation that exists in MEN2 patients, gene sequencing is invaluable in MEN2 syndromes. Indeed the mutations can now be grouped into high (codons 634, 883, 918 and 922), intermediate (codons 611, 618 and 620) and low (codons 609, 630, 768, 790, 791, 804 and 891) risk mutations depending on the age of progression from MTC *in situ*/C-cell hyperplasia to invasive MTC [9]. These data can be used for screening at-risk individuals as well as guiding the treatment of *RET* mutation carriers. Cure can indeed only be achieved in MEN2 patients when the surgical treatment is prophylactic and guided by the result of genetic testing, rather than the clino-biochemical criteria used previously [10].

It is recommended that first-degree relatives of *RET* mutation MEN2 carriers should be genetically tested to establish their status and therefore implement a tailored treatment and surveillance programme. The chance of detecting a *RET* germline mutation in an apparently sporadic MTC ranges between 1% and 7%. The broad range is explained by the significant influence of youth and the presence of multifocality within the thyroid specimen, each of which independently increases the probability of detecting a germline mutation [11]. Genetic testing therefore is appropriate in all patients with apparently sporadic MTC, given the potential benefit of early clinical and surgical intervention both for the patient and affected relatives. The same applies to sporadic phaeochromocytomas which it is now recognised have a genetic cause in well over the often quoted 10% [12].

Clinical picture and management

MEN1

Whilst MEN1 syndrome comprises almost two dozen different endocrine and non-endocrine disease combinations (Table 1) it is most commonly a combination of hyperparathyroidism (in almost 100%), pancreatoduodenal tumours (in up to 80%) and pituitary tumours (in up to 50%). Some patients will not manifest all three classic conditions during their lifetime, so it is sufficient to have two of the three associated diseases to warrant the label of MEN1, and one first-degree relative with at least one condition to have familial MEN1. Carriers of MEN1 gene mutation should be reviewed clinically and biochemically annually in order to detect the manifestations of disease and prevent its adverse consequences.

Parathyroid disease

MEN1 is responsible for up to 4% of primary hyperparathyroidism (1°HPT) in the community. This is typically the presenting feature of MEN1 syndrome and tends to occur several decades prior to the peak incidence associated with sporadic 1°HPT. Virtually all carriers of a MEN1 gene mutation will have biochemical evidence of 1°HPT by the age of 50 years [13, 14]. The disease is almost universally multiglandular, making pre-operative localisation studies in primary surgery irrelevant since a four- gland exploration is mandatory. Pre-operative imaging indeed may be misleading since asymmetry in the size and hyperfunction of the glands is not uncommon.

Whilst it is universally agreed that the surgical treatment of MEN-related 1°HPT is best left in the hands of surgeons with a broad experience of this

Table 1. Expressions of MEN1 with estimated penetrance at 40 years.

Endocrine features

Hyperparathyroidism (90%)

Neuroendocrine GI tumour
- Gastrinoma (40%)
- Insulinoma (10%)
- Non-functioning (20%)
- Others, e.g. VIPoma, somatostatinoma (2%)

Foregut carcinoid
- Thymic carcinoid (2%)
- Bronchial carcinoid (2%)
- Gastric enterochromaffin tumour (10%)

Anterior pituitary tumour
- Prolactinoma (20%)
- Others inc GH, PRL (5%)
- ACTH (2%)
- TSH (rare)

Adrenal cortex
- Non-functioning adenomas (25%)

Non-endocrine features

Facial angiofibromas (85%)
Collagenomas (70%)
Lipomas (30%)

disease, the optimal timing and surgical strategy are the subject of debate. The objective of surgical treatment is to arrest or prevent end organ damage whilst limiting the morbidity and adverse sequelae of surgery. One option is a total parathyroidectomy and cervical thymectomy, which virtually eliminates the risk of HPT recurrence. However, a total parathyroidectomy comes at the price of hypoparathyroidism, which in a young population may be troublesome and expose the patients to the risk of early onset cataracts, calcification of the basal ganglia and adynamic bone disease. In view of this it is desirable to leave a young MEN1 patient with some residual parathyroid function, whether in the form of a forearm parathyroid auto-transplant or by leaving a small vascularised parathyroid fragment marked *in situ* in the neck. The authors prefer this latter option since the graft success rate and the risk of a neoplastic-type growth in the brachioradialis muscle adds unpredictability to the patients' long-term course. Whichever form of residual parathyroid is left, this approach exposes the patient to a risk of recurrent disease in later years.

Pancreatic and enteroneuroendocrine tumours

As many as 80% of MEN1 patients have enteropancreatic islet tumours at autopsy but most are small and non-functional. Significantly fewer have clinical or biochemical manifestations of the disease. Manifestations most commonly include hormonal hypersecretion, most frequently of gastrin from small muticentric enteropancreatic lesions. The clinical presentation of a gastrinoma is Zollinger-Ellison syndrome: atypically located or multiple gastric ulcers or intestinal perforation secondary to the increased acid secretion associated with gastrin excess. Gastrinomas in this context are not only multiple but are frequently associated with other enteropancreatic tumours [15]. Other substances produced include insulin, chromogranin A and B, pancreatic polypeptide, glucagon, somatostatin, serotonin and calcitonin. Less frequently the tumours are few and non-functioning, but all present an unpredictable malignant potential [16]. Overall, however, about 50% of all enteropancreatic lesions have metastasised by the time of diagnosis and up to a third of patients ultimately die of their neuroendocrine malignancy [17].

The diagnosis and localisation of these tumours requires a multidisciplinary approach involving endocrinologists, nuclear medicine, conventional and interventional radiology as well as endoscopic ultrasound for the purposes of localisation of the disease. Surgery, increasingly in the form of a laparoscopic enucleation, is the universally accepted treatment for insulinomas. In contrast most other hypersecretion syndromes can be treated medically in the first instance. The indications and timing of surgery broadly divide the endocrine surgical community into 'doves' and 'hawks', particularly in the asymptomatic patient. Some groups advocate early intervention ranging from enucleation of the pancreatic head and duodenal tumours accompanied by a distal pancreatectomy to a Whipple's pancreatoduodenectomy [18]. The more conservative approach is to avoid prophylactic surgery, working on the principle that cure is difficult to achieve and therefore reserving the complex surgery only for patients with lesions that are either at least 3cm in diameter or showing features of progression.

Pituitary tumours

The prevalence of pituitary tumours in MEN1 syndrome, like the hormonal hypersecretion, varies greatly between series and environments. Most pituitary lesions are under 1cm in diameter (microadenomas) and can secrete a wide range of hormones (Table 1), so annual screening by an endocrinologist with an interest in pituitary disease and review by a pituitary multidisciplinary team is mandatory. Occasionally, however, the pituitary disease can be of considerable volume and cause visual field defects (Figure 1). The treatment issues in pituitary tumours in the MEN context do not differ from sporadic pituitary disease and range from drug treatment (dopamine agonists for prolactinomas) to surgery and radiotherapy for Cushing's disease or acromegaly and for the larger, locally compressive disease that does not respond to medication.

Other manifestations of MEN1

Non-functioning adrenal tumours have been incidentally identified in as many as 40% of MEN1 patients, a feature which may at least in part be related to the frequency of cross-sectional imaging in this group [18]. Up to 14% of MEN1 patients present with neuroendocrine/carcinoid gut tumours. The peculiarity in these patients is that there is a predominance of foregut (thymus, bronchial tree, oesophagogastric and pancreatoduodenal) lesions in contrast to sporadic carcinoids that have a predominantly midgut location.

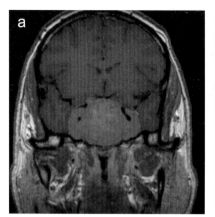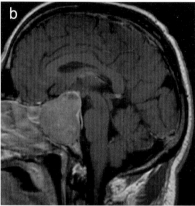

Figure 1. MRI of a large pituitary tumour presenting with a bitemporal hemianopia. a) Coronal view. b) Sagittal view.

MEN2

Over 90% of all MEN2 patients will at some stage have medullary thyroid cancer (MTC) and this is usually the first manifestation of disease. MEN2A accounts for over 75% of MEN2 syndrome and 50% of these patients will at some stage have a phaeochromocytoma and up to a third experience primary hyperparathyroidism [19]. Some rarer MEN2 variants manifest only MTC (familial MTC) or are associated with cutaneous lichen amyloidosis or Hirschsprung's disease (Table 2).

MEN2B is clinically the most aggressive variant of MEN2 syndrome and is characterised by an early onset and a phenotypically aggressive MTC usually accompanied by ganglioneuromatosis and the absence of hyperparathyroidism. The mortality of this disease is significantly higher than in MEN2A due to the MTC, but the phaeochromocytoma risk appears similar.

Medullary thyroid cancer

MTC has an overall incidence of one per million per year, of which MEN2 may be responsible for up to half [20]. MTC is usually the first manifestation of MEN2 and the most likely to cause morbidity and death. Calcitonin, produced by the parafollicular cells, acts as a tumour marker

Table 2. MEN2 syndromes.

	Clinical features in addition to MTC
MEN2A	Phaeochromocytoma Primary hyperparathyroidism
Familial MTC	None
MEN2A with cutaneous lichen amyloidosis	As MEN 2A with trunk lichen amyloidosis
MEN2A with Hirschsprung's disease	Hirschsprung's disease either with full MEN 2A or FMTC alone
MEN2B	Phaeochromocytoma Intestinal, upper airway and mucosal ganglioneuromatosis Marfanoid habitus

that increases in step with the progression from C-cell hyperplasia, localised MTC and MTC metastases, although this increase is not linear. The arrival of the calcitonin assay reduced the disease-specific MTC mortality from 20% to less than 5% and the combination of genetic screening and optimal therapy may bring the life expectancy of these patients towards that of the normal population [21].

The management of MTC in MEN2 patients is dependent upon the presentation which may be clinically evident MTC, a raised calcitonin in the absence of clinical disease or as a consequence of genetic screening. The gathering of genotype-phenotype information is increasingly allowing prophylactic treatment in the form of surgery that can be timed to optimise the chances of cure. The prevailing view is that to achieve cure in MEN2 patients, thyroid surgery should be performed before the age of one year, five years and ten years for high, intermediate and low risk patients, respectively, although counselling of parents of such young children can be challenging in this respect. Both C-cell hyperplasia and MTC are characteristically multicentric involving both lobes so when surgery is performed a total thyroidectomy is mandatory.

Lymph node metastasis is frequent in both the central and lateral neck as well as the mediastinal compartments. In symptomatic disease or disease detected by basal or stimulated calcitonin elevation, the combination of the clinical picture, mutation involved, calcitonin level and age of the patient, guide the appropriate extent of lymph node surgery that aims to control local disease and improve survival. The commonest germline abnormality found in MEN2A is a codon 634 mutation, and large series suggest that no lymph node metastases are present under the age of 14 years of age. In contrast, codon 918 mutations, most frequently associated with MEN2B, are associated with MTC at the age of one year and lymph node metastases under the age of two years, which can guide the extent of surgery in such cases [11]. In the presence of gross cervical lymphadenopathy surgical cure is unlikely, but a prolonged survival in the presence of the disease is not uncommon, so the primary aim of lymphadenectomy is to reduce the morbidity of the local cervico-mediastinal disease.

Phaeochromocytoma

Prior to the advent of genetic screening the mortality from sudden death, especially in pregnancy, secondary to undiagnosed phaeochromocytoma was significant. The genetic diagnosis of MEN2 allows the biochemical screening of MEN2 patients with 24-hour urinary catecholamine and metanephrine assays in mutation carriers. Patients with raised urinary catecholamine and metanephrines can then be imaged using a combination of meta-iodobenzylguanidine (MIBG) scans and cross-sectional imaging to localise the source of the hypersecretion (Figures 2 and 3). Bilateral adrenal disease may be synchronously or metachronously present in as many as 50% of MEN2 patients (Figure 4). Following alpha and beta-blockade, unilateral adrenal phaeochromocytomas can be treated with a unilateral laparoscopic adrenalectomy even if the tumours are of a large size [22]. Bilateral disease can be treated with a bilateral laparoscopic adrenalectomy or with a total adrenalectomy on one side and a cortex-sparing operation contralaterally [23].

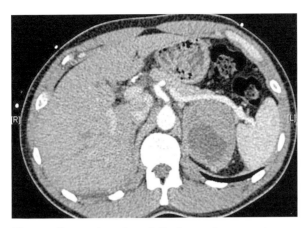

Figure 2. CT of a 7.2cm left phaeochromocytoma.

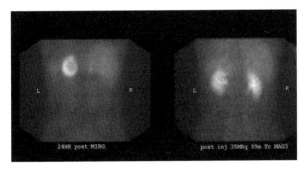

Figure 3. MIBG scan of the patient in Figure 2.

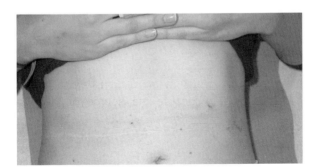

Figure 4. Metachronously presenting phaeo-chromocytomas: two weeks following left laparoscopic adrenalectomy. Right adrenalectomy performed prior to introduction of minimal access approach.

Neither of these approaches is without hazard since adrenal insufficiency can be life-threatening and the long-term sequelae of a subtotal adrenalectomy in this scenario are unknown.

Hyperparathyroidism

Hyperparathyroidism affects up to a third of patients with MEN2 and is commonest in codon 634 mutations [24]. The hyperparathyroid disease has less penetrance than in MEN1 and it presents later and may be caused by single gland disease. Like most 1°HPT seen today it is usually asymptomatic. Screening for the disease with regular corrected serum calcium and parathyroid hormone measurements allows an early diagnosis and treatment prior to evidence of end organ damage that includes renal stone disease and osteoporosis.

The treatment for MEN2-related HPT is a parathyroidectomy which differs from sporadic disease only in that a focused or minimally invasive approach is contraindicated due to the significant risk of multiple gland disease. In most cases, however, the management of parathyroid disease is a problem that presents at the time of the thyroidectomy for prevention or cure of the MEN2-related MTC. In this scenario, the surgical strategies adopted vary from a total parathyroidectomy with or without parathyroid auto-transplantation to a subtotal (*in situ*) parathyroidectomy to remove only macroscopically abnormal glands. Ideally, normal parathyroid glands left *in situ* at the time of the original thyroid surgery should be marked with a non-absorbable marker such as a clip or inert suture material. Whatever the procedure adopted, the results are best when performed by a surgeon with experience in the management of this disease.

The future

MEN syndromes have represented the earliest examples of genetically determined inheritable disease combinations. Whilst much data have been accumulated there remain gaps in our knowledge that will be filled as new mutations are identified and the explanation of the differing penetrance of known mutations becomes clearer. This will allow further optimal tailored care to each affected individual, ideally prior to clinical disease expression.

Key points

- The optimal outcome in patients with MEN syndromes involves the use of genetic testing.

- MEN1 syndrome is caused by a germline mutation of a tumour suppressor gene and leads most typically to the combination of hyperparathyroidism, pituitary tumours and neuroendocrine tumours.

- All patients presenting with primary hyperparathyroidism under the age of 30 years should be considered for MEN1 genetic screening with or without a gut hormone and pituitary hormone screen.

- Both affected and unaffected first-degree relatives of known MEN1 patients should be considered for genetic testing.

- MEN2 syndrome comprises MEN2A, MEN2B and FMTC and is an autosomal dominant hereditary syndrome caused by a germline mutation in the *RET* proto-oncogene.

- All patients diagnosed with MTC should be screened for a phaeochromocytoma prior to surgery and be counselled for *RET* mutation analysis.

- Screening first-degree relatives of MEN2 mutation carriers is mandatory since the genotype-phenotype correlation makes prophylactic surgery possible.

References

1. Underdahl LO, Woolner LB, Black BM. Multiple endocrine adenomas. *J Clin Endocrinol Metab* 1953; 13: 20-47.

2. Wermer P. Genetic aspects of adenomatosis of endocrine glands. *Am J Med* 1954; 16: 363-71.

3. Hayles AB, Kennedy RJL, Bearhs OH, *et al*. Management of a child with thyroid carcinoma. *JAMA* 1960; 173: 21-8.

4. Sipple JH. The association of phaeochromocytoma with carcinoma of the thyroid gland. *Am J Med* 1961; 31: 163-66.

5. Steiner AL, Goodman AD, Powers SR. Study of a kindred with phaeochromocytoma, medullary thyroid carcinoma, hyperparathyroidism and Cushing's disease: multiple endocrine neoplasia, type 2. *Medicine* (Baltimore) 1968; 47: 371-409.

6.   Larsson C, Skogseid B, Oberg K, *et al.* Multiple endocrine neoplasia type 1 gene maps to chromosome 11 and is lost in insulinoma. *Nature* 1988; 332: 85.

7.   Poisson A, Zablewska B, Gaudray P. Menin interacting proteins as clues towards the understanding of multiple endocrine neoplasia type 1. *Cancer Lett* 2003; 189; 1-10.

8.   Marx SJ, Agarwal SK, Kester MB, *et al.* Multiple endocrine neoplasia type 1: clinical and genetic features of the hereditary endocrine neoplasias. *Recent Prog Horm Res* 1999; 54: 397-439.

9.   Machens A, Niccoli-Sire P, Hoegel J, *et al.* Early malignant progression of hereditary medullary thyroid cancer. *N Engl J Med* 2003, 349: 1517-27.

10. Lips CJM. Clinical management of the multiple endocrine neoplasia syndromes: results of a computerised opinion poll at the Sixth International Workshop on Multiple Endocrine Neoplasia and von Hippel-Lindau disease. *J Intern Med* 1998; 243: 589-94.

11. Eng C, Mulligan LM, Smith DP, *et al.* Low frequency of germline mutations in the Ret proto-oncogene in patients with sporadic medullary thyroid carcinoma. *Clin Endocrinol* (Oxf) 1995; 43: 123-7.

12. Neumann HP, Bausch B, McWhinney SR, *et al.* Germ-line mutations in nonsyndromic pheochromocytoma. *N Engl J Med* 2002; 346(19): 1459-66.

13. Trump D, Farren B, Wooding C, *et al.* Clinical studies of multiple endocrine neoplasia type 1 (MEN1). *QJM* 1996; 89(9): 653-69.

14. Uchino S, Noguchi S, Sato M, *et al.* Screening of the *MEN1* gene and discovery of germ-line and somatic mutations in apparently sporadic parathyroid tumours. *Cancer Res* 2000; 60: 5553-7.

15. Norton JA, Fraker DL, Alexander HR, *et al.* Surgery to cure the Zollinger-Ellison syndrome. *N Engl J Med* 1999; 341: 635-44.

16. Le Bodic M-F, Heymann M-F, Lecompte M, *et al.* Immunohistochemical study of 100 pancreatic tumours in 28 patients with multiple endocrine neoplasia type 1. *Am J Surg Pathol* 1996; 20: 1378-84.

17. Pipeleers-Marichal M, Somers G, Willems G, *et al.* Gastrinomas in the duodenums of patients with multiple endocrine neoplasia type 1 and the Zollinger-Ellison syndrome. *N Engl J Med* 1990; 322: 723-7.

18. Skogseid B, Oberg K, Eriksson B, *et al.* Surgery for asymptomatic pancreatic lesions in multiple endocrine neoplasia type 1. *World J Surg* 1996; 20: 872-7.

19. Eng C, Clayton D, Schuffenecker I, *et al.* The relationship between specific RET proto-oncogene mutations and disease phenotype in multiple endocrine neoplasia type 2. International RET mutation consortium analysis. *JAMA* 1996; 276: 1575-9.

20. Ponder BA, Smith D. The MEN II syndromes and the role of the *RET* proto-oncogene. *Adv Cancer Res* 1996; 70: 179-222.

21. Dralle H, Gimm O, Simon D, *et al.* Prophylactic thyroidectomy in 75 children and adolescents with hereditary medullary thyroid cancer: German and Austrian experience. *World J Surg* 1998; 22: 744-50.

22. Ippolito G, Palazzo FF, Sebag F, *et al.* Safety of laparoscopic adrenalectomy in patients with large pheochromocytomas: a single institution review. *World J Surg* 2008; 32(5): 840-4.

23. Lairmore TC, Ball DW, Baylin SB, *et al.* Management of phaeochromocytomas in patients with multiple endocrine neoplasia type 2 syndromes. *Ann Surg* 1993; 217: 595-601.

24. Schuffenecker I, Virally-Monod M, Brohet R, *et al.* Risk and penetrance of primary hyperparathyroidism in multiple endocrine neoplasia type 2A families with mutations at codon 634 of the *RET* proto-oncogene. Groupe d'etude des tumours a calcitonine. *J Clin Endocrinol Metab* 1998; 83: 487-91.

Chapter 10

Neurofibromatosis

Meena Upadhyaya PhD FRCPath
Professor of Medical Genetics and Consultant Molecular Geneticist
Institute of Medical Genetics, Cardiff University, Cardiff, UK

Background

Neurofibromatosis Type 1 (NF1 [MIM 162200]), first described by von Recklinghausen in 1882, is an inherited complex multi-system disorder. This common autosomal dominant disease, with a birth incidence of 1 in 3,500 and a prevalence of one in 5,000 worldwide, is fully penetrant by the age of five years, and exhibits a ten-fold higher mutation rate than most other disease genes [1-4].

Genetics

NF1 gene

The NF1 gene is a large human gene spanning approximately 300kb of 17q11.2, which contains 61 exons, four of which are alternatively spliced, that encode a 12kb mRNA transcript (Figure 1) [2]. Three unrelated genes, OMG, EVI2B and EVI2A, are embedded within the ~61kb intron 27b of the gene. The NF1 gene is an ubiquitously expressed gene, with its protein product, neurofibromin, present at low levels in most tissues but at increased levels in the brain and central nervous system. Neurofibromin exhibits GTPase-activating activity (GAP activity) towards cellular Ras proteins, with the GAP-related domain (GRD), encoded by exons 21-27a, being the most highly conserved region.

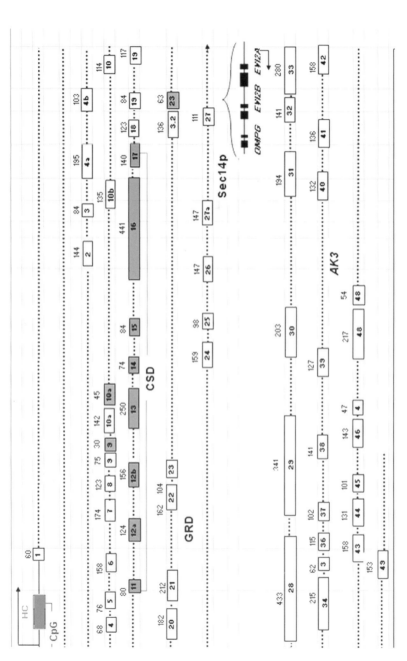

Figure 1. *NF1* gene. Each of the 61 exons are shown (rectangle). The four alternatively spliced exons (9a, 10a-2, 23a, 48a) are identified. The introns are shown by dotted lines. Exons that encode for three recognised domains in neurofibromin are indicated: CSD, GRD and Sec14p. The three embedded genes in intron 27b (*OMG*, *EVI2A* and *EVI2B*) are indicated. An arrow indicates the opposite direction of transcription.

Germline mutations of the *NF1* gene

The *NF1* gene exhibits a high mutation rate, with approximately one mutation per 10,000 gametes per generation, that results in almost half of all mutations being *de novo* events [1]. The identification and characterisation of *NF1* gene mutations continues to be a challenging task, due mainly to the large gene size, the paucity of recurrent mutations, no obvious clustering of mutations, the great diversity of mutation types, and the presence of several highly homologous *NF1* pseudogenes on other chromosomes. At least 1,000 different germline *NF1* mutations have been identified (http://www.hgmd.org), of which the majority (over 80%) are predicted to be truncating lesions.

For non-synonymous missense mutations, 5-10% of all point mutations, it is often difficult to predict pathogenicity in the absence of appropriate functional tests. About a third of all *NF1* mutations are shown, or predicted, to result in aberrations of mRNA splicing, with several nonsense mutations of the gene also resulting in exon skipping [5]. Other coding region mutations disrupting exonic splicing enhancers have also recently been recognised and may cause the exon skipping associated with some of the nonsense and missense mutations of the gene. No mutations have been detected in the *OMG*, *EVI2B* and *EVI2A* genes in any NF1 patients.

Some 5% of NF1 patients exhibit large 1.4Mb genomic deletions that remove the entire *NF1* gene, along with a variable number of the 14 flanking genes (Figure 2). This common 1.4Mb deletion is flanked by a pair

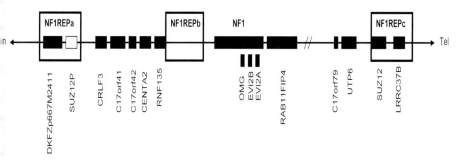

Figure 2. The 14 genes immediately flanking the *NF1* gene within the 1.4Mb deletion region. Genes are indicated by shaded boxes with their gene symbols.

of highly paralogous sequences that facilitate unequal homologous recombination. A less common 1.2Mb deletion also occurs that results from homologous recombination between the *SUZ12* (*JJAZ1*) gene and its pseudogene [6]. The *SUZ12* (*JJAZ1*) gene and pseudogene are completely encompassed within the 1.4Mb deletion.

New *NF1* mutations, especially point mutations, exhibit a bias towards being of paternal origin, while large genomic deletions are usually of maternal origin [2].

NF1 pseudogenes

More than 30 unprocessed *NF1* pseudogene sequences on different chromosomes (2q12-13, 12q11, 14p11-q11, 15q11.2, 18p11.2, 21p11-q11 and 22p11-q11) have been identified by FISH (fluorescence *in situ* hybridisation) analysis with *NF1* cDNAs, and by comparative analysis of the published human genome sequence.

Neurofibromin: the NF1 gene product

Neurofibromin is a large (2818 amino acids) ubiquitously expressed protein, present only at low levels in most tissues with the highest levels found in the CNS, often in association with tubulin. Neurofibromin exhibits structural and amino acid sequence similarity to a large family of evolutionarily conserved proteins, the mammalian GTPase activating proteins (GAP-related proteins) [7]. The most highly conserved region of neurofibromin is indeed the NF1 GAP-related domain (GRD), that is encoded by exons 20-27a. The functional role of the NF1-GRD is the stimulation of the intrinsic GTPase activity of GTP-bound Ras proteins (GAP activity). This GAP activity downregulates activated Ras proteins, and loss of functional neurofibromin in different cell types leads to a loss of growth control in these cells. Activation of Ras is achieved via GTP-binding and the subsequent conformational change involved in the protein. Increased Ras-GTP not only leads to increased signalling through the MAPK (mitogen-activated protein kinase) pathway but also protects cells from apoptosis by activating protein kinase B/Akt via phosphoinositide

3_OH kinase (PI3 kinase). Ras is a key factor of many growth factor signalling pathways and in the absence of neurofibromin it is constitutively activated, resulting in increased cell proliferation and survival.

Increased Ras activity may also be associated with NF1-related learning deficiencies, where it is suspected of leading to long-term potentiation impairment resulting from increased GABA (gamma-aminobutyric acid) mediated inhibition.

The mTOR (mammalian target of rapamycin) signalling pathway was recently shown to be highly regulated in neurofibromas, with the mTOR pathway activated in the absence of growth factors in both NF1 tumours and neurofibromin-deficient cultured cells.

Neurofibromin is also known to interact with a number of other proteins, including tubulin, kinesin, protein kinases A and C, syndecan, caveolin and the amyloid precursor protein, although the biological significance of these interactions is largely unknown. This diversity of protein associations does emphasise, however, that neurofibromin has many other functions than just being a GAP protein.

While the loss of neurofibromin, and the concomitant elevation in activated Ras-GTP levels, may possibly explain tumour formation in NF1, it does fail to account for many of the other clinical features, such as short stature and scoliosis associated with this disorder.

Tumour suppression mechanism

NF1 is a tumour suppressor gene, with the initial constitutional heterozygous inactivating mutations represented by either an inherited or a *de novo* germline mutation. Subsequent somatic inactivation of the normal *NF1* allele is known to be critical for tumour development, although the involvement of additional modifier genes has been suggested. Evidence for large deletions of tumour DNA involving the *NF1* locus, has been found in dermal, spinal and plexiform neurofibromas, malignant peripheral nerve sheath tumours (MPNSTs), phaeochromocytomas, gastrointestinal stromal tumours (GISTs), leukaemia and glomus tumours.

It has been shown that it is only the Schwann cells which carry somatic *NF1* mutations [8] and that tumours only develop when NF1 inactivation in Schwann cells is combined with *NF1* heterozygosity in the tumour environment [9]. There is a clear need to decipher the underlying genetic and biological mechanisms affected by such inherited and acquired *NF1* gene variants, that result in development of benign and malignant tumours in NF1. Few studies have, however, attempted to fully characterise the spectrum of somatic *NF1* mutations present in the various different tumour types of NF1.

Genotype-phenotype associations

Currently, only two established genotype-phenotype correlations have been reported in human NF1. The first involves NF1 patients with large genomic deletions as their germline *NF1* mutation, with such patients often presenting with a more severe disease status, often with a high burden of dermal neurofibromas that develop at an earlier age. Many have dysmorphic features, and also often develop learning disabilities [10]. More importantly, such patients with deleted *NF1* (also referred to as microdeletion patients) exhibit an increased risk of developing malignancy, especially MPNST. This genotype-phenotype association has, however, been recently challenged. We know that about 5% of NF1 patients have a microdeletion, either the common 1.4Mb deletion (a Type I deletion), present in about half the cases, or a 1.2Mb deletion (a Type II deletion), found in almost 40% of the remaining patients. Many of these deletion mutations are found in a mosaic state in patients, with almost 90% of all Type II deletions being identified as mosaic deletions in a recent study. As might be expected from mosaic expression of such deletion mutations, none of these patients exhibited either facial dysmorphism or mental retardation, and they all generally presented with a milder disease phenotype. Microdeletion NF1 patients with atypical deletion sizes have been identified but it is not clear whether larger deletions confer a more severe phenotype and whether certain inherited haplotypes modulate this phenotype.

The second genotype-phenotype association relates to a much more specific mutation, a three base pair deletion within the *NF1* gene, that is correlated with the complete absence of neurofibroma developments in affected patients [11]. The presence of a deletion involving three nucleotides (AAT) in exon 17 of the *NF1* gene is also associated with a much milder NF1 phenotype in many patients, but the most striking finding is the complete absence of cutaneous, subcutaneous, or superficial plexiform neurofibromas in this group. Given that cutaneous neurofibromas are a hallmark clinical feature of NF1, a better understanding of why they fail to develop in all such adult patients should help to identify the underlying pathobiological mechanisms involved in neurofibromagenesis. This AAT deletion results in the loss of a single methionine residue in the mutant neurofibromin and it has been suggested that this might function as a hypomorphic allele. An assessment of the biological effect of this mutation on the protein is urgently required as this observation has clinical importance.

Animal models of NF1

Mouse models of human disease are often developed to help decipher the effects of disease genes on the early development and in trying to establish the underlying mechanisms of development and tumour formation. In NF1, a number of mouse models have been generated that are allowing us to better understand the biology of the disease [7].

Heterozygous mice (*Nf1*[+/-]) do not develop any neurofibromas, hallmark features of NF1, although these mice do exhibit a decreased learning ability, performing poorly in tests of spatial learning and memory. In contrast, homozygous (*Nf1*[-/-]) mice are severely affected and all die *in utero* between days 11.5 and 14 of gestation, usually with severe malformation of the developing heart.

Mice have also been produced in which the *NF1* gene is inactivated either in specific cell types, and/or during specific developmental time windows and these mouse models reflect many of the phenotypic features observed in human NF1 patients. Mice in which multiple genes are inactivated in addition to the murine *Nf1* gene, have also been developed; these models have provided us insight into the interaction of the *NF1* gene with other genes to develop NF1 pathology. Mouse models have enhanced our understanding of NF1 biology and offer a new platform for evaluating therapies for NF1 tumours prior to launching clinical trials.

Clinical picture

The cardinal clinical features of NF1 are dermal pigmentary changes (café-au-lait [CAL] spots and skinfold freckling), dermal neurofibromas and Lisch nodules of the iris.

Neurofibromas

Neurofibromas are benign tumours of peripheral nerve sheath origin (Figure 3), that develop as discrete cutaneous or subcutaneous growths, as well as larger spinal and plexiform tumours. Neurofibromas are mainly comprised of Schwann cells, along with fibroblasts, perineurial cells, mast cells and axons. Dermal neurofibromas normally develop during adolescence, but may occur in patients as young as seven years, and are present in the vast majority of adult NF1 patients. A reported increase in neurofibroma number and size during puberty and pregnancy indicate that hormonal factors can contribute to their growth. Subcutaneous or nodular neurofibromas, located beneath the skin, can be painful when palpated and may undergo malignant change. They are reported to be present in more than a quarter of patients.

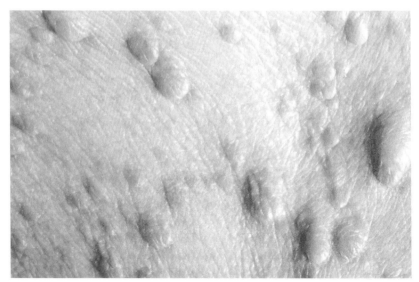

Figure 3. Cutaneous neurofibromas in an NF1 patient.

Plexiform neurofibromas

Much larger plexiform neurofibromas (PNF) are the other main benign tumour type, being present in 30-50% of NF1 patients [12]. These congenitally-developing tumours usually develop in and along the major nerve tracts, often involving multiple fascicles and nerve branches. Almost half of all PNFs are large, extensive tumours, whose growth rate and the pattern of development are difficult to predict.

Three tumour sub-types are recognised, superficial, displacing and invasive PNFs, mainly based on radiological appearances. Superficial PNFs are large, often disfiguring cutaneous or subcutaneous tumours, often asymmetric and diffuse in shape, and have no clear demarcating borders. Usually located immediately above the epifascial membrane, they do not penetrate the underlying musculature. Displacing PNFs are tumours primarily associated with the main nerve trunks, usually having smooth, well-defined margins, and which can compress and displace, but not penetrate, adjacent tissues. In contrast, invasive PNFs present as large diffuse tumours, lacking any defined border, that often penetrate and become deeply embedded among the surrounding tissues.

Malignant peripheral nerve sheath tumours

Individuals with NF1 carry a 7-13% lifetime risk of developing a MPNST that normally arise either from pre-existing PNF, or a focal subcutaneous neurofibroma [13]. MPNSTs are aggressive tumours that often metastasize extensively. These tumours are rarely observed in children with NF1.

Other tumours

Several other tumour types are also associated with NF1, including optic and cerebral gliomas, GISTs, phaeochromocytomas, glomus tumours and leukaemias. These different tumours occur at different frequencies during the lifespan of the patient with NF1 (Table 1).

Table 1. Age-dependent development and frequency of NF1 clinical features.

Disease feature	Age of onset	Frequency (%)
Café-au-lait spots	0-5yrs	>99
Lisch nodules	>3yrs	90-95
Skinfold freckling	>3yrs	85
Cutaneous neurofibromas	>7yrs	>95
Sub-cutaneous neurofibromas	>12yrs	30-40
Spinal neurofibromas	Lifelong	30
Plexiform neurofibroma - visible	Birth onward	30
Plexiform neurofibroma - deep-seated	Birth onward	25
Malignant peripheral nerve sheath tumours	5-75yrs	10
Scoliosis	0-18yrs	10
Pseudarthrosis	0-3yrs	2
Sphenoid wing dysplasia	Birth	1
Bowing or thinning of long bone cortex	Birth	1
Renal artery stenosis	Lifelong	2
Optic pathway glioma	0-7yrs	15
Cerebral glioma	Lifelong	2-3
Juvenile myelomonocytic leukaemia	0-18	<1%
Phaeochromocytoma	>10yrs	2
Duodenal carcinoid	>10yrs	1.5
Gastrointestinal stromal tumours	Lifelong	2.2
Glomus tumours	Adult	1
Macrocephaly	Birth	45
Learning difficulties	Birth	50
ADHD	Birth	38
Epilepsy	Lifelong	7

Other features

Many additional clinical features are also associated with NF1, including various skeletal abnormalities (skeletal and orbital dysplasia, tibial bowing or pseudoarthrosis and scoliosis, sphenoid wing dysplasia, aqueduct stenosis and macrocephaly, and pectus excavatum), cardiovascular abnormalities (artery stenosis), and learning disability and attention deficit (Table 1). The time of onset and severity of most NF1 clinical features are strongly age-dependent and often extremely variable, even within affected families carrying the same *NF1* mutation. CAL spots, PNF and tibial dysplasia are typically recognised within the first year of life.

Variants of NF1

Autosomal dominant multiple café-au-lait spots
An increasing number of families are reported in which affected individuals exhibit a few NF1-like clinical features in two or more generations. Perhaps the best defined are families who only exhibit CAL spots, sometimes in association with skinfold freckling; while some of these autosomal dominant CAL families do show linkage to the *NF1* locus, several others are unlinked.

Familial spinal neurofibromatosis
This is a rare autosomal dominant condition with only two families so far described, with one linked to the *NF1* locus and the other not. The 17q11.2-linked family satisfies several NF1 diagnostic criteria, presenting with multiple spinal neurofibromas and more than six CAL spots. None of those affected exhibited cutaneous neurofibromas, Lisch nodules or any axillary freckling.

Watson syndrome
This syndrome, first described in 1967, is linked to the *NF1* locus. Affected individuals exhibit pulmonary stenosis and learning problems, but very few, if any, cutaneous neurofibromas.

LEOPARD syndrome
This syndrome is characterised by a complex of clinical features, including multiple lentigines, ocular hypertelorism, electrocardiographic

conduction abnormalities, pulmonary stenosis, abnormal genitalia, retardation of growth and sensorineural deafness. While the majority of LEOPARD syndrome cases have either *PTPN11* or *KRAS* mutations, a few cases have been identified with *NF1* missense mutations.

Segmental neurofibromatosis Type 1 (SNF1)

Segmental neurofibromatosis Type 1 (SNF1) is characterised by a regionally-limited distribution of NF1 features, with only one unilateral body segment being involved in most patients, some displaying only pigmentary changes or dermal neurofibromas, and others having both features. Some SNF patients may present with a bilateral symmetrical or asymmetrical involvement of the affected body regions. The SNF1 form of the disorder is not infrequent, with approximately one per 40,000 or 0.02% of the general population affected [14]. The majority of reported cases are, however, sporadic, and the associated clinical phenotype can be quite variable.

Ras pathways and its association with NF1-like syndromes

An increasing number of germline mutations in genes involved in the ever-expanding Ras signalling pathway have now been identified as the underlying cause of several different developmental disorders. These include Noonan, Costello, cardio-facio-cutaneous (CFC), LEOPARD syndromes, capillary arteriovenous malformation, gingival fibromatosis 1, as well as the previously mentioned familial CAL NF1-like disorder caused by *SPRED1* gene mutations (see Figure 4).

Many of the clinical features associated with these syndromes overlap to some extent with NF1. The identification of *NF1* germline mutations in NF1 first indicated that aberrant Ras signalling might contribute to the pathogenesis in some developmental disorders; however, it is the recent identification in Noonan syndrome patients of mutations involving many different genes in the Ras pathway, that now include the *PTPN11*, *SOS1*, *BRAF*, *CRAF*, *KRAS* and *MEK1* genes, that has led to recognition of the Ras pathway developmental syndromes [15]. In LEOPARD syndrome, patients again show some NF1-like features, and mutations of the *SHP2* and *CRAF* genes have been found, while some Costello syndrome patients have *HRAS* mutations. Then in CFC syndrome, mutations of the *SOS1*,

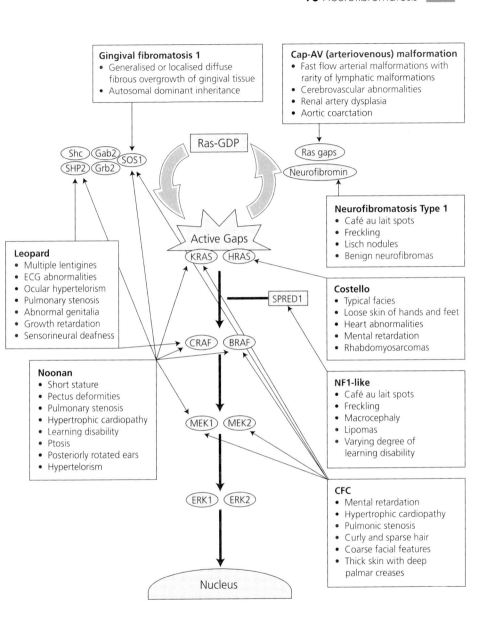

Figure 4. Clinical syndromes associated with mutations in genes of the RAS-MAPK pathway. The syndromes may have overlapping clinical features and multiple genes in the pathway may be mutated in different syndromes.

A guide to cancer genetics in clinical practice

BRAF, KRAS, MEK1 and *MEK2* genes are present. Mutations in the *SPRED1* gene which maps to the Ras pathway and also downregulates Ras activity has very recently been identified in a few NF1-like families who exhibit CALs, skinfold freckling and macrocephaly [16].

Given this plethora of recent research data it seems highly likely that mutations in others within the Ras signalling pathway may well confer an NF1-like phenotype, and/or underlie other developmental syndromes. It will be interesting to discover what degree of commonality of molecular pathology underlies these Ras pathway-related developmental syndromes.

Other types of neurofibromatoses

Neurofibromatosis Type 2 (NF2)

NF2 has a birth incidence of about one in 30,000[17] and is characterised by occurrence of bilateral vestibular schwannomas. The *NF2* gene is located on chromosome 22 (22q12) and encodes the merlin protein [17]. It functions as a tumour suppressor in the pathogenesis of NF2-associated tumours and schwannomas. Individuals with loss-of-function *NF2* mutations such as frameshifts tend to have earlier onset and a more severe disease than do individuals with missense or some splicing mutations. Interestingly, NF2 patients with whole gene deletions tend to have milder manifestations.

Schwannomatosis

Schwannomatosis has only recently been described as a distinct disorder, despite the recent estimates that its incidence is similar to that of NF2 (1 in 30,000). Individuals with schwannomatosis should not fulfil the diagnostic criteria of NF2 or have any of the following features: a vestibular schwannoma on MRI, constitutional *NF2* mutation or a first-degree relative with NF2 [17]. This disorder is autosomal dominantly inherited with variable expression and is linked to a separate locus on chromosome 22. Patients with schwannomatosis develop multiple schwannomas in many regions but not on the vestibular nerve. No other tumours or different clinical manifestations occur in affected individuals. Recently, mutations in *SMARCB1* gene at 22q11 have been identified in a few schwannomatosis families. The protein encoded by this gene is involved in chromatin cell cycle, growth and regulation.

Diagnosis

Genetic testing

While the initial diagnosis is almost always made on a clinical basis, additional specialist examination is often needed for those NF1 children who present with no major disease complications, and who often represent the first case in the family. It is such families who may be especially aided by the identification of a specific *NF1* gene mutation [18].

Early diagnosis of the disease is considered essential so that patients and their families can be offered appropriate counselling, and the affected children can be regularly monitored for complications, such as learning difficulties, optic glioma and hypertension. There has been little demand to date for prenatal diagnosis, possibly because most couples would want to know the clinical severity of the disease in their baby, which currently cannot be predicted. Despite this lack of demand, there is still an urgent need for a cost-effective, rapid and accurate DNA-based test for NF1, and development of a suitable pre-implantation test for NF1 has been reported. The absence of any obvious clustering of mutations within the *NF1* gene clearly necessitates screening of the entire gene for mutations. Furthermore, no single mutation detection test system is currently able to identify the entire spectrum of *NF1* mutations, which includes everything from point mutations through single and multiple exon lesions up to 1.4Mb genomic deletions.

Diagnostic criteria

The consensus NF1 diagnostic criteria were established in 1987 at a National Institutes of Health (NIH) conference in Bethesda (USA) (Figure 5). They include the presence of the following features:

- Six or more café-au-lait spots (>5mm in greatest diameter) in prepubertal patients and (>15mm) in postpubertal individuals.
- Two or more neurofibromas of any type, or one plexiform neurofibroma.
- Freckling in the axillary and/or inguinal regions.
- Optic glioma.

A guide to cancer genetics in clinical practice

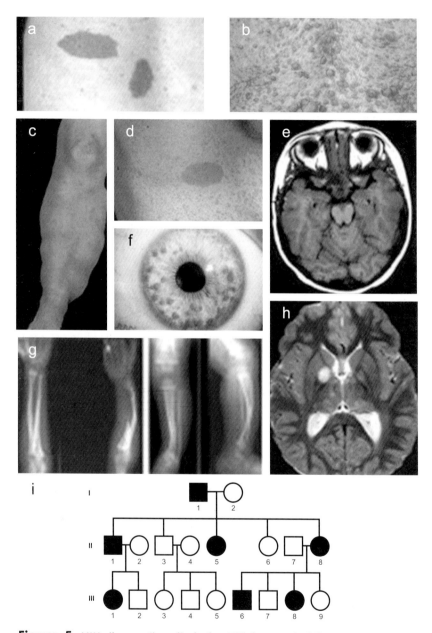

Figure 5. NIH diagnostic criteria for NF1 (agreed at the NIH consensus conference in 1987): a) CAL spots; b) Cutaneous NF; c) PNF; d) Skinfold freckling; e) Optic glioma; f) Lisch nodules; g) Thinning and bowing of long bone cortex; h) Sphenoid wing dysplasia; i) First-degree relative.

- Two or more Lisch nodules (iris hamartomas).
- Distinctive osseous lesions, such as sphenoid dysplasia or thinning/bowing of the long bone cortex with or without pseudarthrosis.
- A first-degree relative (parent, sibling, or offspring) with NF1 defined by the above criteria.

However, clinicians have recently suggested that these diagnostic criteria require updating in light of recent research [19]. A number of NF1-like conditions are now recognised, in which affected individuals exhibit some of these diagnostic criteria. For example, a few families whose only NF1 symptoms were inherited CAL spots, sometimes in association with skinfold freckling, and with no detectable *NF1* mutations, have recently been found to have *SPRED1* gene mutations [16]. Furthermore, in mismatch repair deficiency families, those rare affected individuals who either have homozygous, or compound heterozygous mutations of one or more of their mismatch repair genes, may exhibit a few NF1-like features, usually CAL spots and skinfold freckling. Such individuals, as well as their affected siblings with the same biallelic mismatch repair gene mutation, normally have unaffected parents, and may develop a few large CAL spots that satisfy the NF1 diagnostic criteria, although no germline *NF1* gene mutations are present. It is perhaps worth noting that CAL spots in NF1 usually have a regular outline and uniform depth of pigmentation, whereas CAL spots in patients with mismatch repair gene mutations, and also some individuals with chromosome 17 ring chromosomes, often exhibit irregular margins and pigmentation [19].

The recent improvements in *NF1* mutation detection techniques have led to the suggestion that the presence of a pathogenic *NF1* mutation should now also be included as one of the diagnostic criteria for this disorder.

Clinical management

Genetic counselling

Genetic counselling in NF1 is greatly impeded by the marked intra- and inter-familial variation in NF1 disease expression observed in patients [20].

The combination of this clinical variability and the extensive mutational heterogeneity in NF1, often necessitating labour-intensive mutation screening, means that attempts to produce genotype-phenotype correlations for this disorder are still very much in their infancy. Due to the variability of clinical expression in NF1, disease progression and severity cannot be readily predicted.

When counselling young sporadic cases who present with at least five CAL spots, it has been suggested that an initial molecular testing of these children for the three base pair deletion of exon 17 and *SPRED1* mutation should be considered. However counselling juvenile sporadic cases will also be difficult especially if this represents a segmental NF1 case.

Clinical management

The clinical management of children with NF1 is still complex due to the diversity and age-related presentation of many symptoms. NF1 children therefore require yearly appraisal of development and education, and a physical examination of skin, spine, blood pressure, height and weight and head circumference. Visual testing should be done until the age of seven. Clinical management for NF1 patients requires a multidisciplinary approach and the use of multi-specialties in the NF1 clinic is required. Surgical intervention can also be offered in certain cases. There is no current successful treatment for any symptoms and regular clinical surveillance is required.

Potential therapies

Any protein found to be involved in NF1 tumorigenesis may be a potential target for future therapies. Thus, the Ras signal pathway has been targeted with Ras-GTP levels being increased in both benign and malignant tumours. Farnesyl transferase (FT) was found to be critical in anchoring the Ras protein to the cell membrane and is required for *RAS* function [19]. Treatment with FT inhibitors has shown an inhibition of growth in NF1-deficient MPNST cell lines; however, although these FT inhibitors decreased hyperproliferation, they had little effect on the invasion in neurofibromin-deficient Schwann cells. They also failed to have any significant effects on PNF. This is an antifibrotic tissue growth antagonist that modulates actions of several cytokines including PDGF, FGF, EGF, intracellular adhesion molecule and TGFB1. It is used to inhibit the growth-promoting effects of fibroblasts.

Imanitib, a tyrosine kinase inhibitor, has been used with some success in patients with metastatic pylocytic astrocytomas. The use of rapamycin in preclinical studies, as well as early clinical studies in humans, has yielded promising results.

Mice heterozygous for *NF1* mutations have also been identified to have some degree of learning problems and it was found that reduction in Ras activity improves this deficiency. It has been found that treatment with levostatin has shown improved learning ability by inhibiting the p21 Ras activity. Levostatin has also been used to treat skeletal dysplasia in animals. NF1 is a good example of a human disease gene model where successful cloning of the gene has resulted in enhanced basic and translational research and in clinical trials.

The future

Because of the difficulty in detecting *NF1* mutations, it is critical to develop better *NF1* mutation detection techniques that allow high throughput and are cost effective and both sensitive and specific. A high resolution oligonucleotide-based *NF1* microarray that provide a complete coverage of the *NF1* gene is in development and should be available for molecular diagnosis in the near future.

Identification of additional consistent genotype-phenotype relationships would offer improved genetic counselling and predictive testing for NF1 patients, and identification and characterisation of modifying loci would help us to better understand how NF1 pathology may be associated with interactions of different loci.

The development of better surgical and imaging techniques to manage this complex group of patients is urgently needed.

In order to improve basic knowledge of the biological mechanisms involved in NF1, the development of better *in vitro* cell culture and NF1 animal models would be useful.

Key points

♦ The three neurofibromatoses, designated as NF1, NF2 and schwannomatosis, all exhibit complex phenotypes associated with both tumour and non-tumour manifestations. NF1 is the commonest form of these disorders.

♦ NF1 is an autosomal dominantly inherited disorder with almost complete penetrance by five years of age.

♦ Both the time of onset and severity of most NF1 clinical features are strongly age-dependent as well as being variable, even within families that carry the same *NF1* gene mutation.

♦ Molecular diagnosis is based on *NF1* mutation analysis; however, the uptake for the prenatal diagnosis is quite limited because the severity of the disease cannot be predicted in any affected fetus.

♦ In the absence of a successful treatment for NF1, regular clinical surveillance and appropriate genetic counselling are warranted, especially for younger affected patients.

References

1. Huson S, Hughes R. *The neurofibromatoses: A pathogenetic and clinical overview.* London: Chapman & Hall Medical, 1994: 487.
2. Upadhyaya M, Cooper DN. *NF1: From genotype to phenotype.* Oxford: BIOS Publishers, 1998.
3. Friedman JM, Gutmann DH, Riccardi VM. *Neurofibromatosis: phenotype, natural history and pathogenesis*, 3rd ed. Baltimore: Johns Hopkins University Press, 1999: 400.
4. Korf BR, Rubenstein. *A handbook for patients, families and healthcare professionals.* New York: Thieme Med Publ, 2005: 253.

5.   Messiaen LM, Wimmer K. *NF1* mutational spectrum. In: *Neurofibromatoses.* Kaufmann D, Ed. *Monogr Hum Genet* 2008; 16: 63-77.

6.   Kehrer-Sawatzki H. Structure of the *NF1* gene region and mechanisms underlying gross *NF1* deletions. In: *Neurofibromatoses.* Kaufmann D, Ed. *Monogr Hum Genet* 2008; 16: 89-102.

7.   Chichowski K, Jacks T. *NF1* tumour suppressor gene function. Narrowing the GAP. *Cell* 2000; 104: 593-604.

8.   Serra E, Rosenbaum T, Winner U, *et al.* Schwann cells harbor the somatic *NF1* mutation in neurofibromas: evidence of two different Schwann cell subpopulations. *Hum Mol Genet* 2000; 9: 3055-84.

9.   Zhu Y, Ghosh P, Charnay P, *et al.* Neurofibromatosis in NF1: Schwann cell origin and role of tumour environment. *Science* 2002; 296: 920-2.

10.   Kayes LM, Burke W, Riccardi VM, *et al.* Deletions spanning the neurofibromatosis 1 gene: identification and phenotype of five patients. *Am J Hum Genet* 1994; 54: 424-36.

11.   Upadhyaya M, Huson SM, Davies M, *et al.* A complete absence of cutaneous neurofibromas associated with a 3-bp in-frame deletion in exon 17 of the *NF1* gene (c.2970_2972 del AAT): a clinically significant genotype-phenotype correlation? *Am J Hum Genet* 2007; 80: 140-51.

12.   Ferner RE, Huson SM, Thomas N, *et al.* Guidelines for the diagnosis and management of individuals with neurofibromatosis 1. *J Med Genet* 2007; 44: 81-8.

13.   Evans DG, Baser ME, McGaughran J, *et al.* Malignant peripheral nerve sheath tumours in neurofibromatosis 1. *J Med Genet* 2002; 39: 311-4.

14.   Ruggieri M, Huson SM. The clinical and diagnostic implications of mosaicism in the neurofibromatoses. *Neurology* 2001; 56: 1433-43.

15.   Nyström AM, Ekvall S, Berglund E, *et al.* Noonan and cardio-facio-cutaneous syndromes: two clinically and genetically overlapping disorders. *J Med Genet* 2008; 45: 500-6.

16.   Brems H, Chmara M, Sahbatou M, *et al.* Germline loss-of-function mutations in *SPRED1* cause a neurofibromatosis 1-like phenotype. *Nat Genet* 2007; 39: 1120-6.

17.   McClatchey AI. Neurofibromatosis. *Ann Rev Pathol Mech Dis* 2007; 2: 191-216.

18.   Griffiths S, Thompson P, Frayling I, *et al.* Molecular diagnosis of neurofibromatosis type 1: 2 years experience. *Fam Cancer* 2007; 6: 21-34.

19.   Huson SM. The neurofibromatoses: classification, clinical features and genetic counselling. In: *Neurofibromatoses.* Kaufmann D, Ed. *Monogr Hum Genet* 2008; 16: 1-20.

20.   Gutmann DH, Aylsworth A, Carey JC, *et al.* The diagnostic evaluation and multidisciplinary management of neurofibromatosis 1 and neurofibromatosis 2. *JAMA* 1997; 278: 51-7.

Chapter 11

Familial gastric cancer

Vanessa Blair BHB MBChB
Surgical Research Fellow
Department of Surgery, University of Auckland, Auckland, New Zealand

Susan Parry FRACP
Gastroenterologist
New Zealand Familial Gastrointestinal Cancer Registry, Auckland City Hospital and Department of Gastroenterology, Middlemore Hospital, Auckland, New Zealand

Background

Historically, Napoleon Bonaparte is probably the most famous case of familial gastric cancer described. While familial aggregation is relatively common in gastric cancer, occurring in 10-15% of cases, in low incidence countries less than 5% of cases display an autosomal dominant inheritance pattern [1]. The first description of a molecular basis for hereditary gastric cancer was in a large New Zealand Maori family (family A) with an extensive history of gastric cancer, where a detailed pedigree facilitated a genetic linkage analysis resulting in detection of the first germline mutation in the E-cadherin gene (*CDH1*) in 1998 [2]. With the identification of further mutations, Guilford *et al* proposed that *CDH1* germline mutations define a hereditary cancer syndrome dominated by diffuse gastric cancer, called hereditary diffuse gastric cancer (HDGC) [3]. Despite extensive mutation searching in other candidate genes, no further mutations have been found in families where gastric cancer predominates.

Genetics

The *CDH1* gene codes for epithelial-cadherin, a calcium-dependent cell-to-cell adhesion molecule that is a key component of adherens junctions between epithelial cells. E-cadherin is central to development, cell differentiation and the maintenance of tissue integrity, complex core processes that are tightly regulated. Absent or reduced E-cadherin function due to somatic *CDH1* mutation is known to parallel invasion and metastasis in many sporadic carcinomas, but has only been reported as an early event in sporadic diffuse gastric cancer and lobular breast cancer [4]. Exactly how E-cadherin loss or down-regulation initiates gastric cancer is not known, although a model has been proposed whereby HDGC carcinogenesis is initiated by loss of E-cadherin in the gastric stem cell compartment [5].

To date 70 different *CDH1* mutations have been reported in 87 different HDGC families, but have never been detected in families with intestinal gastric cancer [6]. The first *CDH1* founder mutation was recently reported in four families from Newfoundland, Canada [7]. The ethnicity of HDGC families is diverse, although it is notable only eight are from Asia. Given the high incidence of sporadic gastric cancer in Asian populations, chance clusters of sporadic gastric cancer may obscure the identification of the families with inherited susceptibility.

Germline *CDH1* mutations are spread relatively evenly throughout the gene, with 70% truncating and 30% missense mutations [6]. Although the truncating mutations clearly abrogate normal E-cadherin function, the functional significance of missense mutations is not straightforward. Cell aggregation and invasion assays have been developed to evaluate the effect of *CDH1* missense mutations and when combined with other parameters, missense mutations can be divided into pathogenic and neutral variants to guide genetic counselling [8, 9].

Penetrance

In a study of 11 of the first HDGC families identified, the cumulative risk estimate for advanced gastric cancer by 80 years was 67% in men and 83% in women with wide confidence intervals (Table 1) [10]. Mean age at diagnosis was 40 years. While no firm evidence exists for variable penetrance, initial data raise this possibility (Table 1) [2, 7].

Table 1. Penetrance of gastric and breast cancer in HDGC.

HDGC family/s	Cancer (cases)	Cumulative risk (95% CI)	Mean age onset	Reference
11 HDGC families (includes family A)	Stomach (n=80)	67% in males (33-99%) 83% in females (58-100%) by age 80 years	40y (range 14-85y)	10
Family A	Stomach (n=25)	70% by age 60 years	35y (range 14-74y)	2
Newfoundland family	Stomach (n=29)	40% in males (12-91%) 63% in females (19-99%) by age 75 years	not stated	7
11 HDGC families	Breast (n=7)	39% in females (12-84%) by age 80 years	53y (range 39-64y)	10
Newfoundland family	Breast (n=16)	52% in females (29-94%) by age 75 years	not stated	7

Clinical picture

Gastric cancer

The hallmark of early HDGC is the presence of multiple foci of signet-ring cell carcinoma confined to the superficial lamina propria (TNM stage T1a) with no nodal metastases (Figure 1) [11-13]. In at-risk family members identified to have a disease-causing *CDH1* mutation, prophylactic gastrectomy is the only way to completely eliminate the risk of developing gastric cancer. When examined, these gastrectomy specimens nearly always appear macroscopically normal as the microscopic HDGC foci typically lie beneath an intact surface epithelium with minimal alteration to pit pattern. However, complete pathological mapping of these specimens as part of a research protocol reveals a wide variation in the number of T1a foci (range 1 to 487) and no stomach has been identified without early carcinoma [1, 13, 14].

Pathological mapping of 19 gastrectomy specimens from New Zealand families has revealed there is a greater density of foci which are typically larger in the transitional zone between body and antral type mucosa (Figure 1) and the antrum is usually spared [1, 13]. This has ramifications for endoscopic screening but it should be noted that this pattern has not been

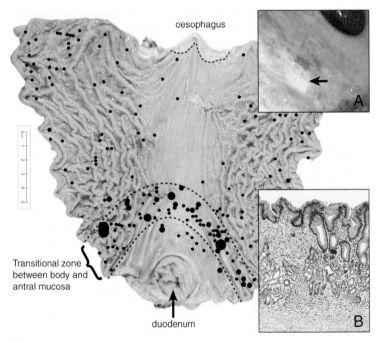

Figure 1. Gastrectomy specimen from a 28-year-old *CDH1* mutation carrier showing distribution of microscopic foci of early signet-ring cell carcinoma (black dots to scale, except foci <2mm shown as 2mm for visibility). Clustering of foci (including largest foci) is seen in the transitional zone. Inset A: pale area seen at chromoendoscopy in transitional zone, biopsy carcinoma. Inset B: H&E stained section showing edge of focus of early HDGC - signet-ring cells infiltrate beneath normal epithelium on left, normal mucosa on right.

detected in the other HDGC mapping study [14] and given that 16 of the 19 stomachs studied were from family A, a genotype-phenotype correlation is possible.

In advanced stages, HDGC is indistinguishable from advanced sporadic diffuse gastric cancer. In HDGC gastrectomy series the average age at surgery is 32 years and the presence of T1a carcinoma in all (100%) stomachs contrasts markedly with the estimated penetrance for advanced HDGC at the same age which is 4% [10]. Even allowing for an extended time lag for progression from these early HDGC foci, the penetrance for advanced HDGC at 50 years is still only 21% in men and 46% in women [10]. These observations suggest that a prolonged indolent phase may occur before stage T1a HDGC foci invade beyond the mucosa; however, the duration of this indolent phase is unpredictable [1].

Breast cancer

The only other malignancy known to occur in HDGC families at an elevated frequency is breast cancer, but lifetime cumulative risk estimates are limited by small numbers: 39% in 11 HDGC families with seven cases [10] and 52% in one HDGC family with 16 cases [7] (Table 1). Evidence suggests it is the lobular form of breast cancer that is associated with HDGC. While breast cancer histotype has been confirmed in only 21/75 cases in HDGC families, 18/21 (86%) were lobular, in contrast to sporadic breast cancer where 10% are lobular. Furthermore, three mutation carriers from different HDGC families have been described with metachronous lobular breast cancer and diffuse gastric cancer [1].

Other cancers

Colorectal, prostate and other cancers have been documented in HDGC families, but not at frequencies significantly above the risk of the general population [10]. Two cases of signet-ring carcinoma of the colon have been reported in HDGC families [15, 16].

Diagnosis and surveillance

Diagnosis

Current classification systems for familial gastric cancer are not entirely satisfactory. A practical approach is to apply the framework depicted in Figure 2 when patients present to clinic. This framework draws on the International Gastric Cancer Linkage Consortium (IGCLC) criteria originally proposed in 1999 [17], including suggested modifications [15] and consensus of the New Zealand HDGC Group [1]. Once it has been established that the affected family members are all on the same side of the family (i.e. paternal or maternal) the next step is to determine histotype - is it diffuse or intestinal gastric cancer? This terminology derives from the Lauren classification, which acknowledges a distinction between gastric carcinomas where gland formation is evident, called 'intestinal' type and 'diffuse' gastric cancer, where it is not [18]. Diffuse gastric cancer has discohesive, isolated cells with diverse morphologies, which may include signet-ring cells [18]. Advances in molecular biology have associated the diffuse phenotype with absent, reduced or abnormal E-cadherin expression.

Once histotype is known, the next step is to see if the family history fits either IGCLC or modified criteria (Figure 2). In families with intestinal gastric cancer, criteria differ slightly depending on the incidence of gastric cancer in the background population. If the incidence is high, the criteria are analogous to the Amsterdam criteria in HNPCC [17]. No mutations have been identified in familial intestinal gastric cancer (FIGC) families, and management is guided by assessment of risk based on each family history.

In families with confirmed diffuse gastric cancer in at least one family member, depending on the criteria fulfilled, screening for germline *CDH1* mutation may be appropriate (Figure 2). The two original IGCLC criteria for diffuse gastric cancer families were either two confirmed cases of diffuse gastric cancer in first or second-degree relatives, with the diagnosis being made in one under 50 years, or three confirmed cases of diffuse gastric cancer at any age. Modifications to these criteria (1A and 2A in Figure 2) have been proposed to allow for the fact that it is often not possible to confirm histotype in more than one family member [15]. Families meeting criteria 1, 1A, 2, or 2A should be offered *CDH1* mutation testing as a mutation will be found in 30-50% of such families [15, 16].

Diffuse gastric cancer families with a confirmed *CDH1* mutation need to be distinguished from families with familial diffuse gastric cancer (FDGC) where no *CDH1* mutation has been identified because of the different management implications. To allow this, it has been proposed that the term HDGC be reserved only for those families with a confirmed *CDH1* mutation and this nomenclature will be used here [1]. A rare autosomal dominant syndrome characterised by gastric hyperplastic polyps and diffuse gastric cancer has been reported, in which no *CDH1* mutations have been identified, an entity distinct from HDGC [19].

While a family history of gastric cancer is present in 10-15% of gastric cancer patients, in low incidence countries only 5% or less will have a history suggesting autosomal dominant inheritance [1]. It has been estimated HDGC may account for 1% or less of all cases of gastric carcinoma, with the incidence likely to be even lower among high-risk populations like Japan, where less than 1% of cases have an autosomal dominant pattern [1].

Additional criteria have been suggested (criteria 3 to 6, Figure 2) that broaden the clinical situations where *CDH1* mutation screening may be appropriate [15].

Gastric cancer in other familial cancer syndromes

Germline mutations in the *KIT* gene have been described in rare families with gastrointestinal stromal tumours (GISTs). GISTs arise from connective tissue, thus are quite separate from gastric carcinoma. Gastric cancer may occasionally occur as part of the tumour spectrum in other familial cancer syndromes (Figure 2).

Genetic testing

Families confirmed to have diffuse gastric cancer and meeting the criteria can be offered testing for *CDH1* mutation; however, for all other families the only 'genetic testing' available is under the auspices of research for new mutations in candidate genes. Searching for *de novo* *CDH1* mutations in young onset 'sporadic' diffuse gastric cancer patients

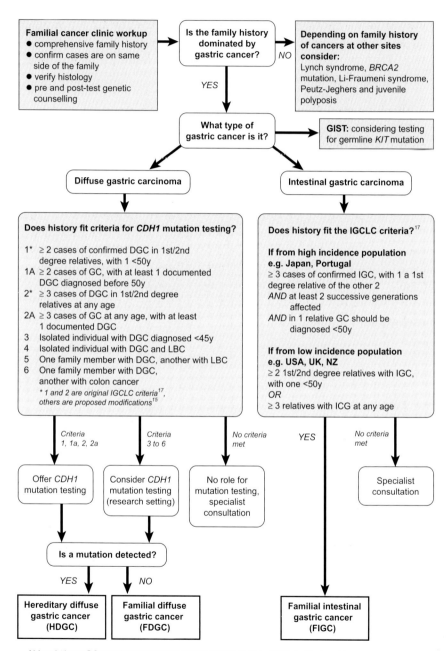

Abbreviations: GC gastric cancer; DGC diffuse gastric cancer; IGC intestinal gastric cancer;
LBC lobular breast cancer; GIST gastrointestinal stromal tumour

Figure 2. Management algorithm for familial gastric cancer.

is controversial because of the low mutation yield, averaging 7% (range 0-20%) across the eight studies in this area to date [20]. Proposed criteria vary, with testing suggested if the individual with diffuse gastric cancer is under 35 or alternatively 45 years of age [8, 15].

There are many factors that need to be considered when counselling HDGC families prior to testing children and adolescents. These include: psychological impact, informed consent, the limitations of surveillance techniques and the morbidity and mortality of prophylactic gastrectomy, but probably the most important is age-related risk. The risk of advanced HDGC in children is very low. In the 87 HDGC families reported, only six (7%) have a case of advanced gastric cancer diagnosed under 20 years and of the six patients, four are from one family in New Zealand, the youngest being a 14-year-old. In the vast majority of HDGC families the youngest patient has been diagnosed in their mid to late twenties or thirties. This family variation has impacted on the guidelines made regarding the age to offer genetic testing, surveillance and prophylactic gastrectomy (Table 2) [1].

Clinical surveillance

Gastroscopy

Gastroscopy is the only technique currently considered as a possible surveillance measure for individuals with a high risk of gastric cancer (Table 2). There are no clinical trials upon which to base recommendations for surveillance in either FIGC or FDGC families and even in HDGC there is only one study on gastroscopic surveillance. On the basis of population screening for gastric cancer in high incidence countries like Japan, annual white-light gastroscopy beginning at an age ten years prior to the youngest case of gastric cancer in the respective family is often advised. However, individuals should be informed of the limitations of such surveillance with regard to detecting gastric cancer at an early stage.

In HDGC the role of surveillance gastroscopy is controversial because diffuse gastric cancer typically infiltrates beneath an intact surface epithelium without producing ulceration or elevation of the mucosa (unlike intestinal gastric cancer). Consistent with this, *CDH1* mutation carriers

Table 2. Management of gastric and breast cancer in HDGC.

Presymptomatic *CDH-1* mutation testing

<14y	Testing children under 14y is usually not appropriate.
14-16y	Consider testing on a case by case basis (see text).
≥16y	All family members should be offered testing.

Surveillance gastroscopy

All patients must be informed there is an unquantifiable risk that carcinoma may be missed at gastroscopy.

Gastroscopy should be performed by specialists with experience in recognising early HDGC lesions (see text).

14-16y   Consider annual gastroscopic surveillance on a case by case basis in mutation carriers.

≥16y   Annual surveillance gastroscopy is recommended until an age when prophylactic gastrectomy is appropriate.

Prophylactic gastrectomy

<16y   The risk of advanced gastric cancer is very low; prophylactic surgery not advised before growth complete.

16-20y   Carcinoma risk <1%; surveillance gastroscopy is usually a more appropriate approach at this age.

20-30y   Carcinoma risk ~4% by 30y; prophylactic gastrectomy is recommended.

Delaying prophylactic gastrectomy beyond this age carries significant risk, but in selected families with a history of late onset HDGC may be appropriate (see text).

Breast surveillance

The limitations of preliminary data on breast cancer risk should be explained.

≥35y   Screening should include 6-monthly breast examination and annual imaging.

Mammography alone is inadequate for screening in HDGC. Ultrasound and preferably MRI are recommended in addition to mammography.

Routine prophylactic mastectomy is not recommended, but may be appropriate in some HDGC families.

who have proceeded to prophylactic gastrectomy have all had normal pre-operative endoscopy despite microscopic foci of early signet-ring cell carcinoma being identified in the resection specimen. Multiple random gastric biopsies taken during surveillance gastroscopy have also failed to detect carcinoma in HDGC [14]. Due to its limitations, surveillance gastroscopy as first-line management is generally only recommended in *CDH1* mutation carriers under the age of 20 years, an age below which prophylactic gastrectomy is not usually recommended for reasons that will be outlined later. Surveillance gastroscopy is also advised in *CDH1* mutation carriers planning prophylactic surgery in their 20s or later and likewise in those who decline prophylactic surgery. In general, surveillance gastroscopy is poorly tolerated in children under 14 years of age. In line with age limits for genetic testing, annual surveillance should usually start at 16 years (Table 2).

In a surveillance series from New Zealand, 33 *CDH1* mutation carriers who declined prophylactic gastrectomy had annual standard endoscopy followed by congo red/methylene blue chromoendoscopy for five years [21]. Chromoendoscopy was an improvement over standard white-light gastroscopy, facilitating detection of 56 'pale lesions' in ten patients, of which 23 (41%) were carcinoma. The pale lesions were 3-10mm, with those highly suspicious for carcinoma having distinct pallor (Figure 1) [21]. Chromoendoscopy has since been discontinued due to new concerns over congo red toxicity but subsequently the two gastroenterologists regularly performing the HDGC endoscopies began detecting pale lesions on standard white-light endoscopy with biopsy proving carcinoma. The experience with chromoendoscopy led to an appreciation that pale areas are visible at standard endoscopy, but as they are so subtle, they would easily be overlooked as 'within normal limits' by most endoscopists. Reliable detection of minute HDGC foci (under approximately 4mm) anywhere in the stomach is probably an unrealistic expectation by either white light endoscopy, chromoendoscopy or perhaps even any of the newer endoscopic surveillance modalities such as confocal endoscopy and narrow band imaging [21].

Breast surveillance
Compared to ductal breast cancer, lobular breast carcinoma is more difficult to detect because of its diffuse growth pattern and relative lack of

microcalcification. While there are no breast screening studies specific to groups at high risk for lobular breast carcinoma, ultrasound is more sensitive than mammography in the detection of sporadic lobular breast carcinoma [1]. Recent evidence suggests MRI is the most sensitive screening modality in high-risk groups generally, although it has a higher false positive rate. Consequently surveillance to detect lobular breast carcinoma in HDGC should include, in addition to mammography, ultrasound and MRI [1]. Surveillance should begin at age 35y and taking the lead from BRCA protocols, should include six-monthly clinical examinations with a yearly interval for radiological screening (Table 2).

Clinical management

Stomach

Total gastrectomy: prophylactic and for screen-detected carcinoma

Currently, prophylactic gastrectomy remains the only option to eliminate an inherited risk of gastric cancer and its role in *CDH1* mutation carriers is well established (Table 2). There are anecdotal reports of prophylactic gastrectomy in families where no mutation has been detected, but generally surveillance gastroscopy would be recommended in this situation.

In the 21st century, the issues surrounding total gastrectomy relate more to its lifelong morbidities than the mortality risk, but the latter cannot be overlooked. Peri-operative mortality after major gastrointestinal surgery is in the range 0-6% in most recent series. However, in young, healthy HDGC patients, when performed by an experienced upper gastrointestinal surgeon, the mortality risk for total gastrectomy is closer to 1% [1]. Broadly, the risk of a *CDH1* mutation carrier developing advanced gastric cancer before age 20 years is approximately matched by the mortality risk of prophylactic gastrectomy. By the age of 18 years in boys and 15 years in girls, 97% have finished height growth and weight increase begins to level off. Since gastrectomy is associated with a reduction in bodyweight, often exceeding 10%, it is likely to compromise growth in teenagers.

Patients need to be fully informed of the long-term consequences of total gastrectomy, reviewed in detail elsewhere [1, 12, 22]. The need for altered meal size, frequency and content can considerably affect lifestyle. The nutritional consequences need full explanation, including the need for life-long vitamin B12 injections. Knowledge regarding the effect of total gastrectomy on female fertility is limited. Given that the pelvic cavity is not disturbed by gastrectomy and providing there are no major postoperative complications, a significant reduction in fertility is unlikely, but must be discussed [1]. All women post-gastrectomy should receive nutritional advice prior to conception, particularly about folate intake.

For the above reasons, prophylactic gastrectomy is not usually recommended in mutation carriers under 20 years [1], the rationale being that the morbidity and mortality risks relating to the surgery outweigh the cancer risk in young patients. While five members of family A have had gastrectomy between 15-19 years, all were diagnosed with early carcinoma by gastroscopic surveillance. It is important to appreciate that the age-related management recommendations in HDGC are guidelines; the age of onset and penetrance in each HDGC family must be taken into account and in some HDGC families with a history of relatively late onset disease, the timing of prophylactic surgery will be influenced accordingly [20].

Staging and choice of operation

Patients with surveillance-detected disease are staged with a CT scan and, if appropriate, also endoscopic ultrasound. D2 dissection with preservation of the spleen and pancreas is the standard operative approach. The controversy surrounding the increased mortality risk versus survival benefit in D2 versus D1 resection for gastric cancer has been subject to extensive review. Evidence suggests that when performed in specialist upper gastrointestinal units, D2 resection without resection of the spleen or distal pancreas confers little, if any, additional risk and would generally be performed in both prophylactic and screen-detected cases, despite the fact that no nodal metastases have been reported in early HDGC [1, 11, 12]. Roux-en-Y oesophagojejunostomy without construction of a jejunal pouch reservoir is the standard approach.

Management of the gastric margins

It is essential to ensure complete resection of the entire gastric mucosa. Determining the exact location of the squamocolumnar junction relative to the anatomical gastro-oesophageal junction is hindered by the lack of a palpable or visible serosal surface marking. One approach is to transect the oesophagus 3-4cm above the anatomical gastro-oesophageal junction and visually confirm an intact cuff of squamous mucosa [1]; this has some advantages over intra-operative frozen section to confirm the margin [22].

Prognosis and follow-up post-gastrectomy

Five-year survival in early gastric cancer is over 90% in almost all Western and Japanese series and in stage T1a approaches 95%. This indicates prognosis in early HDGC will likely be excellent, although long-term survival is currently unknown. It is possible that prophylactic gastrectomy will unmask a risk of carcinoma at other sites. There is no indication for follow-up endoscopy after gastrectomy unless symptoms develop. Follow-up should include review of nutrition, weight, B12 injections and other supplement intake.

Breast

Prophylactic mastectomy may be appropriate in some HDGC families with a strong history of breast cancer and should be considered on a case by case basis. Until penetrance data are more robust, it should not be considered routine in HDGC. Advice from a breast specialist should be sought about tamoxifen prophylaxis and before prescribing oral contraception or hormone replacement therapy.

Chemoprevention and lifestyle advice

There are no trials of chemoprevention in HDGC. General lifestyle advice about known risk factors for sporadic gastric cancer would seem appropriate, such as reducing intake of salted and preserved foods, increasing intake of fresh fruit and vegetables, not smoking and avoiding excessive alcohol. Most HDGC patients have not had *Helicobacter pylori* infection, but if present, it should be eradicated [1].

The future

The management of HDGC has evolved dramatically in the decade since *CDH1* mutations were first described. New endoscopic surveillance modalities need to be explored for those at risk of developing FIGC, FDGC and HDGC. Success is dependent on these modalities being able to identify subtle distortions of the gastric mucosa. Until such time, prophylactic gastrectomy is the only management option that eliminates the risk of gastric cancer in *CDH1* mutation carriers.

Key points

♦ A family history of gastric cancer is present in 10-15% of gastric cancer patients, but in low incidence countries only 5% or less will have a history suggesting autosomal dominant inheritance.

♦ Classification of familial gastric cancer requires verification of histotype: diffuse versus intestinal.

♦ In diffuse gastric cancer families meeting criteria for *CDH1* mutation testing, 30-50% will have a pathogenic germline mutation identified.

♦ Early HDGC is characterised by multiple foci of signet-ring cell carcinoma which typically lie beneath an intact surface epithelium.

♦ The lifetime penetrance for advanced HDGC is 70%.

♦ Surveillance gastroscopy is generally recommended for *CDH1* mutation carriers under 20 years, those planning prophylactic surgery in their 20s or later and patients who decline prophylactic surgery.

♦ Prophylactic gastrectomy is usually recommended between age 20-30 years, but the age of onset and penetrance in each HDGC family must be considered when discussing the timing of prophylactic surgery.

♦ Lobular breast cancer occurs at an increased frequency in HDGC and surveillance is recommended.

References

1. Blair V, Martin I, Shaw D, *et al*. Hereditary diffuse gastric cancer: diagnosis and management. *Clinical Gastroenterology and Hepatology* 2006; 4: 262-75.
2. Guilford P, Hopkins J, Harraway J, *et al*. E-cadherin germline mutations in familial gastric cancer. *Nature* 1998; 392(6674): 402-5.
3. Guilford P, Hopkins J, Grady W, *et al*. E-cadherin germline mutations define an inherited cancer syndrome dominated by diffuse gastric cancer. *Human Mutation* 1999; 14(3): 249-55.
4. Berx G, Becker K, Höfler H, *et al*. Mutations of the human E-cadherin (*CDH1*) gene. *Human Mutation* 1998; 12(4): 226-37.
5. Humar B, Fukuzawa R, Blair V, *et al*. Destabilized adhesion in the gastric proliferative zone and c-Src Kinase Activation mark the development of early diffuse gastric cancer. *Cancer Res* 2007; 67(6): 2480-89.
6. Guilford PJ, Blair V, More H, *et al*. A short guide to hereditary diffuse gastric cancer. *Hereditary Cancer in Clinical Practice* 2007; 5(4): 183-94.
7. Kaurah P, MacMillan A, Boyd N, *et al*. Founder and recurrent *CDH1* mutations in families with hereditary diffuse gastric cancer. *JAMA* 2007; 297(21): 2360-72.
8. Suriano G, Oliveira C, Ferreira P, *et al*. Identification of *CDH-1* germline missense mutations associated with functional inactivation of the E-cadherin protein in young gastric cancer probands. *Human Molecular Genetics* 2003; 12(5): 575-82.
9. Suriano G, Seixas S, Rocha J, *et al*. A model to infer the pathogenic significance of *CDH1* germline missense variants. *J Med Genet* 2006; 84: 1023-31.
10. Pharoah P, Guilford P, Caldas C, *et al*. Incidence of gastric cancer and breast cancer in *CDH1* (E-cadherin) mutation carriers from hereditary diffuse gastric cancer families. *Gastroenterology* 2001; 121: 1348-53.
11. Huntsman DG, Carneiro F, Lewis FR, *et al*. Early gastric cancer in young asymptomatic carriers of germline E-cadherin mutations. *New Engl J Med* 2001; 344(25): 1904-9.
12. Chun YS, Lindor NM, Smyrk TC, *et al*. Germline E-cadherin mutations: is prophylactic gastrectomy indicated? *Cancer* 2001; 92(1): 181-7.
13. Charlton A, Blair V, Shaw D, *et al*. Hereditary diffuse gastric cancer: predominance of multiple foci of signet ring cell carcinoma in distal stomach and transitional zone. *Gut* 2004; 53: 814-20.
14. Carneiro F, Huntsman DG, Smyrk TC, *et al*. Model of the early development of diffuse gastric cancer in E-cadherin mutation carriers and its implications for patient screening. *J Pathol* 2004; 203: 681-87.
15. Brooks-Wilson AR, Kaurah P, Suriano G, *et al*. Germline E-cadherin mutations in hereditary diffuse gastric cancer: assessment of 42 new families and review of genetic screening criteria. *J Med Genet* 2004; 41: 508-17.
16. Oliveira C, Bordin MC, Grehan N, *et al*. Screening E-cadherin in gastric cancer families reveals germline mutations only in hereditary diffuse gastric cancer kindred. *Human Mutation* 2002; 19: 510-7.
17. Caldas C, Carneiro F, Lynch HT, *et al*. Familial gastric cancer: overview and guidelines for management. *J Med Genet* 1999; 36(12): 873-80.

18. Fenoglio-Preiser C, Carneiro F, Correa P, *et al.* Gastric Carcinoma. In: *World Health Organisation Classification of Tumours: Pathology and Genetics, Tumours of the Digestive System.* Hamilton SR, Aaltonen L, Eds. Lyon: IARC Press, 2000: 39-52.
19. Seruca R, Carneiro F, Castedo S, *et al.* Familial gastric polyposis revisited: autosomal dominant inheritance confirmed. *Cancer Genetics & Cytogenetics* 1991; 53: 97-100.
20. Pedrazzani C, Corso G, Marrelli D, *et al.* E-cadherin and hereditary diffuse gastric cancer. *Surgery* 2007; 142(5): 645-57.
21. Shaw D, Blair V, Framp A, *et al.* Chromoendoscopic surveillance in hereditary diffuse gastric cancer: an alternative to prophylactic gastrectomy? *Gut* 2005; 54(4): 461-8.
22. Lewis FR, Mellinger JD, Hayashi A, *et al.* Prophylactic total gastrectomy for familial cancer. *Surgery* 2001; 130(4): 612-9.

Chapter 12

Familial pancreatic cancer

John Windsor FRACS MD
Professor of Surgery
Department of Surgery, University of Auckland, Auckland, New Zealand

Susan Parry FRACP
Gastroenterologist
New Zealand Familial Gastrointestinal Cancer Registry, Auckland City Hospital and Department of Gastroenterology, Middlemore Hospital, Auckland, New Zealand

Background

Pancreatic adenocarcinoma remains one of the most deadly of cancers with an overall five-year survival of less than 5% [1, 2]. Less than a quarter of patients are suitable for a 'curative' resection and less than a quarter of those who undergo such treatment survive five years. Adjuvant chemotherapy has now become the standard of care, but the incremental benefit is only an improvement in five-year survival from 8% to 21% [3]. This dismal outlook will not improve until it is possible to reliably identify individuals at increased risk for earlier diagnosis and treatment [4]. The proof that early detection prolongs life is still wanting.

While the majority of pancreatic adenocarcinoma cases are sporadic, early detection is more likely in those patients with familial pancreatic adenocarcinoma (FPC). It has been commonly stated that FPC is responsible for 10% of cases of pancreatic adenocarcinoma [5]. More recent prospective studies from Sweden and Germany, using strict criteria of confirmation by histology and medical records, suggest that the familial proportion of pancreatic adenocarcinoma is less than that, with a prevalence of only 1.9-2.7% [6, 7].

A family history of pancreatic adenocarcinoma is an important risk factor for developing pancreatic adenocarcinoma, and the risk increases with the number of first-degree relatives with the diagnosis. In a prospective registry-based study, the observed to expected ratio of pancreatic cancer was 4.6 (CI 0.5-16.4) with one affected first-degree relative, 6.4 (CI 1.8-16.4) with two, and 32 (CI 10.2-74.7) with three [8].

It is common for families of patients with pancreatic adenocarcinoma (sporadic or familial) to ask about risk to themselves and other members of the family. There is now a sufficient body of evidence to inform relatives of their relative risk of developing pancreatic adenocarcinoma.

Definition of familial pancreatic cancer

There is no agreed definition of FPC, although the one most widely accepted is individuals with two or more first-degree relatives with pancreatic adenocarcinoma [9] and who are not part of another familial cancer syndrome. The familial aggregation in pancreatic adenocarcinoma is not just due to hereditary predisposition, but is also influenced by variable gene penetrance (not all gene carriers will develop pancreatic adenocarcinoma), environmental factors, family size and chance.

Genetics

There are several clinical syndromes and diseases in which there is a recognised inherited predisposition to pancreatic adenocarcinoma, in addition to FPC. These include hereditary pancreatitis, cystic fibrosis and defined familial cancer syndromes [10] (Table 1), in some of which genetic mutations have been identified and lifetime risk of cancers can been estimated [9].

Table 1. Clinical syndromes and diseases with increased risk of developing pancreatic carcinoma: genetics and lifetime risk.

Syndrome/disease	Gene(s)	Locus	Lifetime risk
Hereditary breast/ovarian cancer	BRCA2	13q	5%
FAMMM syndrome	CDKN2A	9p	19%
Cystic fibrosis	CFTR	7q	25%
Peutz-Jeghers syndrome	STK11	19p	35%
Hereditary pancreatitis	PRSS1, SPINK1	7q, 5q	40%
Lynch syndrome	DNA MMR	2p, 3p	Unknown

FAMMM - Familial Atypical Multiple Mole Melanoma

Familial pancreatic cancer has been considered a genetically heterogeneous disorder caused by mutations in different oncogenes and/or modifier genes, although recent segregation studies suggest that it may be caused by a single major gene [11]. Although the actual FPC gene has not been identified, a FPC susceptibility locus has been mapped to chromosome 4q32-34 in a large kindred with an autosomal dominant inheritance pattern [12]. This is a unique locus, not associated with any of the recognised familial cancer syndromes.

Precursor lesions

Specific genetic alterations accumulate during the progression from histologically normal epithelium to high-grade pancreatic intra-epithelial neoplasia. Each of the key genetic alterations contributes to neoplastic progression and the development of clonal populations and these cells can evolve from non-invasive precursor lesions (pancreatic intra-epithelial neoplasia) labelled PanIN-1a, 1b, 2 and 3 [13].

Environmental risk factors for pancreatic cancer

There are a number of environmental factors that increase the risk of pancreatic cancer in individuals from FPC kindreds. The most important factor is cigarette smoking. It is an independent risk factor, which is more so in males and younger members of FPC kindreds [14]. An interaction between family history and smoking was first reported in 2001 [15,16]. More recent work has determined that smoking increases the risk of pancreatic cancer in FPC four-fold, and that it brings forward the onset of pancreatic cancer by ten years [14]. This is important to note because it influences the timing of when screening should commence. Smoking cessation reverses this risk of pancreatic cancer, but this effect takes more than a decade. Other risk factors, including chronic pancreatitis, are reviewed elsewhere [9,17].

Clinical picture

Patients with FPC usually present with advanced disease. When the adenocarcinoma is in the head of the pancreas, patients often present with obstructive jaundice, and sometimes with pruritus. When in the body and tail of the pancreas the adenocarcinoma usually grows quite large before the onset of non-specific symptoms. It is common for patients to present with lethargy, anorexia and weight loss. The development of dull mid-back pain is a sinister sign and suggests tumour extension beyond the pancreas.

The detection of patients with pancreatic adenocarcinoma prior to the onset of symptoms is the challenge. There are no specific biomarkers in clinical use and existing tumour markers (e.g. CA 19-9 and CEA) do not have a role in screening. The only long-term survivors following resection with or without chemotherapy are those with early stage disease. The best hope of early detection is by surveillance of individuals from FPC kindreds.

Diagnosis and surveillance

The clinical assessment of individuals reporting a family history of pancreatic adenocarcinoma should include a detailed personal and family history to exclude one of the other familial syndromes associated with an increased risk of pancreatic cancer as outlined in Table 1.

Family tree and determining risk

The key step in assessing the risk of pancreatic adenocarcinoma for an individual is the construction of the family tree over at least three generations. If the individual appears to be at an increased risk, then referral to a clinical genetics service is appropriate. Formal pedigree analysis will allow a more accurate assessment of risk and inform discussion regarding surveillance and the role of genetic testing. Referral to an FPC registry can subsequently be facilitated for individuals confirmed to be at increased risk of developing pancreatic adenocarcinoma.

Genetic testing

The current understanding of the genetics of pancreatic cancer has been reviewed [2, 18]. The role of genetic testing is well established in at-risk individuals considered to have one of the recognised familial cancer syndromes (Table 1). The situation is less clear for individuals from FPC kindreds. The current position is that genetic testing outside of controlled studies should be avoided because we do not know the relevant germline mutations in FPC [4]. In some circumstances it may be appropriate, after genetic counselling, for an individual to consent to storage of DNA, for subsequent genetic testing when more is known about the genetics of FPC.

Surveillance

Although there is no established standard that states who should enter a surveillance program, there is general agreement that members of FPC kindreds should be offered surveillance, especially if they smoke and/or have chronic pancreatitis. Similarly there are no established standards for what constitutes an acceptable surveillance protocol [2]. The possible elements include the following:

- ◆ Tumour markers (e.g. CA 19-9 and CEA), but these do not have adequate sensitivity for screening.

- Imaging (e.g. CT, MRI and ultrasound scanning), but these do not have adequate resolution to detect early pancreatic cancer, let alone precursor lesions.

- Endoscopic retrograde pancreatography (ERP), but this is probably too invasive as a primary screening tool. The analysis of pancreatic juice for DNA methylation, DNA mutations, and protein overexpression is an area of active research.

- Endoscopic ultrasonography (EUS) is the most promising modality, but is highly operator-dependent and not widely available outside major centres. EUS can detect quite subtle changes associated with pancreatic intra-epithelial neoplasia, including parenchymal heterogeneity, echogenic foci and hypoechoic nodules.

EUS meets many of the requirements of a screening test being a minimally invasive procedure that is able to detect pancreatic adenocarcinoma before symptoms develop. Proof that EUS screening improves outcome in high-risk individuals is not yet available.

The first screening study from the University of Washington Medical Centre, Seattle, combined both EUS and ERP in testing 35 members of 13 FPC families [19]. There were 12 (34%) individuals with abnormalities, all of whom had a pancreatectomy. An update on this series shows that a total of 15 patients have had a pancreatectomy (12 total, 3 partial) [9]. Histology revealed no invasive cancer, but they were all found to have dysplasia, PanIN II (n=5) and PanIN III (n=10). This group went on to perform a decision analysis on EUS screening [20]. It was concluded that EUS-based screening of FPC kindreds is cost-effective, although the benefit appears to be limited to populations with a pre-test probability of pancreatic dysplasia of 16% or greater and in individuals under 70 years of age. The degree of dysplasia was not specified.

The second important screening study from the Johns Hopkins Medical Institution, Baltimore, and the Mayo Clinic, Rochester, used EUS alone as the screening tool in 38 high-risk asymptomatic individuals [21]. Abnormalities found on EUS were then screened with EUS-guided fine-needle aspiration for cytology, ERP and CT scanning. There were six pancreatic masses identified (one invasive ductal adenocarcinoma, one benign intraductal papillary mucinous neoplasm [IPMN], two serous cystadenomas and two non-neoplastic masses) and seven other incidental symptomatic gastrointestinal findings. Of the six masses, only two were clinically significant pancreatic neoplasia, giving a clinically significant yield of 5% (2/38) or 1:20.

These studies demonstrate that EUS is likely to be the cornerstone of surveillance. There is currently a rapid diffusion of this technology and access to it should become easier. Nevertheless, the skills required for the consistent detection of subtle abnormalities suggest that surveillance of high-risk individuals should be undertaken in major high volume centres, and preferably in association with a genetic service. If access to EUS is impossible, then high quality cross-sectional imaging, by CT or MRI, will need to suffice.

Surveillance guidelines

The following are accepted guidelines for surveillance of high-risk individuals [22]:

* Primary surveillance should be undertaken using EUS after genetic counselling.
* Surveillance should be done in an expert centre, as success is operator-dependent.
* Surveillance should not be done unless pancreatectomy would be considered for dysplasia/early cancer.
* Surveillance is less useful if there is concurrent chronic pancreatitis.
* Surveillance should be initiated at 50 years old or 10 years before the youngest age of diagnosis of pancreatic adenocarcinoma in a family member. If the individual is a smoker then surveillance should be initiated a decade earlier.
* Annual surveillance is reasonable.

Familial pancreatic cancer registries

There are a number of established FPC registries around the world. As well as providing support and education for families, registries provide an important opportunity to evaluate pathogenesis, natural history, biomarkers, genetic predisposition and new diagnosis, treatment and chemoprevention strategies. In addition, knowledge gained from the study of FPC may be useful in improving the diagnosis, management and prognosis of sporadic pancreatic adenocarcinoma. It is important that at-risk individuals from FPC kindreds are offered involvement with an appropriate registry.

Clinical management

It is important to establish a management strategy for detected abnormalities, before embarking on surveillance. There are a number of management options including ongoing surveillance at a shorter interval (e.g. three or six months), cross-sectional imaging (e.g. CT or MRI scanning), ERP (with or without pancreatic fluid cytology), and EUS-guided fine-needle aspiration for cytology. The Washington group has adopted a policy of performing a laparoscopic distal pancreatectomy in order to obtain a tissue diagnosis [23].

Prophylactic pancreatectomy cannot be recommended in asymptomatic high-risk individuals without evidence of dysplastic pancreatic lesions, given the significant morbidity of the procedure and the unknown penetrance in the different settings of FPC [4]. The management of patients with a PanIN II lesion is uncertain, as the natural history remains to be defined. Patients with a PanIN III lesion and no mass could be offered continuing surveillance although a total pancreatectomy is a good option, because of the multifocal and widespread nature of precursor lesions [9]. Patients must be informed of the risks and consequences of total pancreatectomy, but it is a viable option in selected patients. Most pancreatic adenocarcinomas develop in the pancreatic head and if a patient at high risk develops a symptomatic lesion, management would be along orthodox lines [24].

Prevention

The most important preventative measure is to stop smoking and formal assistance should be offered.

The future

Less invasive and more sensitive approaches to surveillance are required. The potential exists in the future for the use of genomic or proteomic biomarker analyses of pancreatic juice, serum, urine or stool samples.

Chemoprevention is a promising concept in this field, but not more than that. When an effective agent is available, genetic testing will assume a critical role in the management of high-risk individuals.

Key points

- The majority of pancreatic adenocarcinoma cases are sporadic, with no known inherited predisposition.
- Recent prospective studies suggest the proportion of pancreatic adenocarcinoma that is familial is less than 3%.
- Family history of pancreatic adenocarcinoma remains the most important risk factor for developing pancreatic adenocarcinoma and increases with the number of affected first-degree relatives.
- Genetic testing in individuals thought to have one of the recognised familial cancer syndromes (Table 1) is recommended, but the situation is much less clear for individuals from FPC kindreds.
- The best chance of reducing the high mortality of pancreatic adenocarcinoma is the identification of high-risk individuals and enrolment into a surveillance program to enable early diagnosis and treatment.
- Endoscopic ultrasonography is the mainstay of screening.
- The most important preventative measure is to stop smoking.
- It remains unproven that early detection of pancreatic adenocarcinoma will prolong life.

References

1. Warshaw A, Fernandez-del Castillo C. Pancreatic carcinoma. *N Engl J Med* 1992; 326(7): 455-65.
2. Konner J, O'Reilly E. Pancreatic cancer: epidemiology, genetics and approaches to screening. *Oncology* 2002; 16(12): 1615-38.
3. Neoptolemos J, Stocken D, Friess H, *et al*. A randomized trial of chemoradiotherapy and chemotherapy after resection of pancreatic cancer. *N Engl J Med* 2004; 350(12): 1200-10.
4. Rieder H, Bartsch D. Familial pancreatic cancer. *Fam Cancer* 2004; 3(1): 69-74.
5. Lynch H, Smyrk T, Kern S, *et al*. Familial pancreatic cancer: a review. *Semin Oncol* 1996; 23(2): 251-75.
6. Hemminki K, Li X. Familial and second primary pancreatic cancers: a nationwide epidemiologic study from Sweden. *Int J Cancer* 2003; 103(4): 525-30.
7. Habbe N, Langer P, Sina-Frey M, *et al*. Familial pancreatic cancer syndromes. *Endocrinol Metab Clin North Am* 2006; 35(2): 417-30.
8. Klein A, Brune K, Petersen G, *et al*. Prospective risk of pancreatic cancer in familial pancreatic cancer kindreds. *Cancer Res* 2004; 64(7): 2634-8.
9. Brentnall T. Management strategies for patients with hereditary pancreatic cancer. *Curr Treat Options Oncol* 2005; 6(5): 437-45.
10. Lynch H, Brand R, Deters C, *et al*. Hereditary pancreatic cancer. *Pancreatology* 2001; 1(5): 466-71.
11. Klein A, Beaty T, Bailey-Wilson J, *et al*. Evidence for a major gene influencing risk of pancreatic cancer. *Genet Epidemiol* 2002; 23(2): 133-49.
12. Eberle M, Pfutzer R, Pogue-Geile K, *et al*. A new susceptibility locus for autosomal dominant pancreatic cancer maps to chromosome 4q32-34. *Am J Hum Genet* 2002; 70(4): 1044-8.
13. Klein W, Hruban R, Klein-Szanto A, *et al*. Direct correlation between proliferative activity and dysplasia in pancreatic intraepithelial neoplasia (PanIN): additional evidence for a recently proposed model of progression. *Mod Pathol* 2002; 15: 441-7.
14. Rulyak S, Lowenfels A, Maisonneuve P, *et al*. Risk factors for the development of pancreatic cancer in familial pancreatic cancer kindreds. *Gastroenterology* 2003; 124(5): 1292-9.
15. Tersmette A, Petersen G, Offerhaus G. Increased risk of incident pancreatic cancer among first-degree relatives of patients with familial pancreatic cancer. *Clin Cancer Res* 2001; 7(3): 738-44.
16. Schenk M, Schwartz A, O'Neal E, *et al*. Familial risk of pancreatic cancer. *J Natl Cancer Inst* 2001; 93(8): 640-4.
17. Hart A, Kennedy H, Harvey I. Pancreatic cancer: a review of the evidence on causation. *Clin Gastroenterol Hepatol* 2008; 6(3): 275-82.
18. Cowgill S, Muscarella P. The genetics of pancreatic cancer. *Am J Surg* 2003; 186(3): 279-86.
19. Rulyak S, Brentnall T. Inherited pancreatic cancer: surveillance and treatment strategies for affected families. *Pancreatology* 2001; 1(5): 477-85.

20. Rulyak S, Kimmey M, Veenstra D, *et al.* Cost-effectiveness of pancreatic cancer screening in familial pancreatic cancer kindreds. *Gastrointest Endosc* 2003; 57(1): 23-9.

21. Canto M, Goggins M, Yeo C, *et al.* Screening for pancreatic neoplasia in high-risk individuals: an EUS-based approach. *Clin Gastroenterol Hepatol* 2004; 2(7): 606-21.

22. Canto M. Screening for pancreatic neoplasia in high-risk individuals: who, what, when, how? *Clin Gastroenterol Hepatol* 2005; 3(7 Suppl 1): S46-8.

23. Rulyak S, Brentnall T. Inherited pancreatic cancer: improvements in our understanding of genetics and screening. *Int J Biochem Cell Biol* 2004; 36(8): 1386-92.

24. Muller M, Friess H, Kleeff J, *et al.* Is there still a role for total pancreatectomy? *Ann Surg* 2007; 246: 966-75.

Chapter 13

Hamartomatous polyposis syndromes

Brandie Heald MS CGC
Certified Genetic Counselor
Center for Personalized Genetic Healthcare, Lerner Research Institute,
Cleveland Clinic, Cleveland, Ohio, USA

Matthew F Kalady MD
Staff Surgeon
Department of Colorectal Surgery, Digestive Disease Institute, Cleveland
Clinic, Cleveland, Ohio, USA

Charis Eng MD PhD FACP
Sondra J and Stephen R Hardis Chair of Cancer Genomic Medicine
Chairman and Director, Genomic Medicine Institute
Director, Center for Personalized Genetic Healthcare, Lerner Research
Institute, Cleveland Clinic, Cleveland, Ohio, USA
Professor and Vice Chairman of Genetics, Case Western Reserve
University School of Medicine, Cleveland, Ohio, USA

Background

The hamartomatous polyposis syndromes are a group of rare autosomal dominant conditions that are characterised by the presence of hamartomatous polyps in the gastrointestinal tract. Included among these disorders are juvenile polyposis syndrome (JPS), Peutz-Jeghers syndrome (PJS), and the PTEN-hamartoma tumour syndrome (PHTS). The PHTS includes Cowden syndrome, Bannayan-Riley-Ruvalcaba syndrome (BRRS), and Proteus syndrome. Each of the hamartomatous polyposis syndromes carries a unique risk for colonic and/or extra-colonic manifestations. Recognition and diagnosis is critical so that appropriate genetic counselling and management can be provided.

Juvenile polyposis syndrome

Juvenile polyposis coli was first described by McColl *et al* in 1964 [1] and is estimated to occur in 1 in 100,000 individuals. Patients with JPS are predisposed to hamartomatous polyps and malignancy in the gastrointestinal tract. 'Juvenile' is indicative of the type of polyp rather than the age of onset. Juvenile polyps possess an abundant lamina propria devoid of smooth muscle and a normal epithelial component. Approximately 2% of children and adolescents will have a solitary juvenile polyp, which does not carry an increased risk of malignancy and is distinct from JPS. Three genes have been associated with JPS: *BMPR1A* located on 10q22.3, *SMAD4* on 18q21.2, and *ENG1* on 9q33-q34.1.

Peutz-Jeghers syndrome

PJS was first reported in 1895 [2], but was not recognised as a distinct entity until 1949 [3]. PJS is characterised by mucocutaneous pigmentation and polyposis of the small bowel. Peutz-Jeghers polyps have a characteristic frond-like structure and appropriate epithelium of the gastrointestinal tract and associated smooth muscle proliferation. Patients with PJS are at increased risk for gastrointestinal and extra-intestinal cancers. PJS is prevalent in 1 in 25,000 to 1 in 280,000 live births. Germline mutations in *STK11* on 19p13.3 have been identified as a susceptibility gene for PJS.

PTEN-hamartoma tumour syndrome

Cowden syndrome was first recognised in 1962. It is one of the few genetic syndromes that was named for the first patient described with the condition, Rachel Cowden. It was nearly ten years later when Bannayan reported the first patient with what later became known as BRRS [4]. The susceptibility locus for Cowden syndrome was mapped to 10q23-q24 in

1996 and, subsequently, germline mutations in *PTEN* were identified in patients and families with Cowden syndrome and in BRRS. PHTS was coined to unify the clinically described syndromes that are caused by germline *PTEN* mutations [5].

Other

In addition to the syndromes described above, hamartomatous polyps have been reported in patients with Gorlin syndrome (nevoid basal cell carcinoma syndrome), hereditary mixed polyposis syndrome, multiple endocrine neoplasia 2B (MEN2B; Chapter 9), and neurofibromatosis type 1 (NF1; Chapter 10).

Gorlin syndrome is characterised by jaw keratocysts and multiple basal cell carcinomas prior to age 30. Macrocephaly, dysmorphic features, skeletal abnormalities, and certain central nervous system, cardiac, and ovarian tumours are key features of this syndrome. Multiple gastric polyposis has been associated with this condition [6]. Gorlin syndrome is caused by germline alterations in *PTCH*.

Hereditary mixed polyposis syndrome was described in a family that developed a variety of types of polyps and carcinoma [7]. Among the family members adenomatous and hyperplastic polyps as well as atypical juvenile polyps were reported. Typically there were fewer than 15 polyps at presentation and no extracolonic disease. Hereditary mixed polyposis was initially mapped to *CRAC1* on 15q13-q14 [7], but this was later questioned when a germline mutation in *BMPR1A* was identified in a similar Chinese family.

Interestingly, ganglioneuromatous polyps are typical of MEN2B and NF1. This type of polyp is amongst the hamartomatous polyps described in Cowden syndrome and BRRS [8]. Therefore, all three syndromes, PHTS, MEN2B and NF1, should be considered in the genetic differential diagnosis of ganglioneuromatous polyps. However, unlike NF1 and PHTS, ganglioneuromatosis of the gut is more typical in MEN2B (as opposed to polyps), typically associated with classic physical stigmata, and virtually all (97-99%) individuals with MEN2B harbour a germline *RET* mutation.

Genetics

Juvenile polyposis syndrome

JPS is believed to be a fully penetrant condition with variable expression. Approximately 60% of cases are familial, while the remaining 40% are believed to occur sporadically [9]. Germline alterations in *SMAD4*, *BMPR1A*, and *ENG1* cause JPS. Prior to the discovery of *BMPR1A* and *SMAD4*, *PTEN* mutations were identified in three patients with so-called JPS. However, upon further scrutiny, it was felt that Cowden syndrome could not be excluded as diagnoses for these patients [10]. It is important to note, moreover, that the manner in which the clinical diagnosis of JPS is made added to this confusion.

SMAD4
SMAD4(MADH4) on 18q21.2 is a tumour suppressor gene in the transforming growth factor beta (TGF-β) signal transduction pathway. Mutations have been identified in six of the eleven exons. Approximately 20% of patients will have detectable *SMAD4* mutations by sequencing [11]. Patients with *SMAD4* mutations have a higher prevalence of giant gastric polyps when compared with patients with *BMPR1A* mutations [12]. Additionally, patients with *SMAD4* mutations have a risk of developing hereditary haemorrhagic telangiectasia (HHT) [13]. HHT is an autosomal dominant condition that is characterised by skin and mucosal telangiectasias, cerebral, pulmonary, and hepatic arteriovenous malformations, and an increased risk of associated haemorrhage. The course of disease in patients with *SMAD4* mutations appears to be similar to patients with HHT without associated JPS.

BMPR1A
BMPR1A located on 10q22.3 is a type I receptor of the TGF-β super family. It regulates bone morphogen protein (BMP) intracellular signalling through *SMAD4*. Sequencing will identify mutations in 20% of cases [11].

ENG1
Recently, two patients with JPS were found to have mutations in *ENG1*, a gene on 9q33-q34.1 previously associated with HHT [8]. Both patients presented with early onset polyposis (ages 3 and 5), but neither had

features of HHT at the time of evaluation. No additional patients have been reported with mutations in this gene.

Peutz-Jeghers syndrome

STK11(LKB1) is composed of ten exons, nine of which are coding. It is a tumour suppressor gene that is unique in that it was the first gene described to result in the loss of catalytic activity of a serine/threonine kinase. Manifestations of the disease are believed to occur because of somatic loss of the second allele. Sequencing will detect 39-69% of mutations. Large deletions account for approximately 30% of mutations. It was originally believed that a second locus exists for PJS, but identification of large deletions within *STK11* refutes this hypothesis.

PJS is believed to have incomplete penetrance with variable expression. Genotype-phenotype correlations have been examined: individuals with missense mutations are more likely to have a later age of polypectomy and presentation of other symptoms when compared with those with truncating mutations and no identifiable mutation.

PTEN-hamartoma tumour syndrome

Cowden syndrome and BRRS are both autosomal dominantly inherited disorders. *PTEN* is a tumour suppressor gene and is the first identified cancer susceptibility gene that encodes a phosphatase. PTEN protein is a dual-specificity/dual-activity phosphatase. Its lipid phosphatase activity signals through the PI3K/AKT pathway and plays an important role in G1 arrest and apoptosis. The AKT pathway is upstream of TSC2/TSC1, proteins encoded by the susceptibility genes of the tuberous sclerosis complex, and of mTOR. PTEN's protein phosphatase activity is now believed to predominate when PTEN is in the nucleus and signalling down the MAPK pathway and eliciting G1 arrest.

Approximately 80% of patients who meet the diagnostic criteria for Cowden syndrome, 60% of patients with BRRS, and 50% with Proteus syndrome will have detectable intragenic mutations. Another 10% of patients with Cowden syndrome will have *PTEN* promoter mutations, and

10% of patients with BRRS will have a deletion within or encompassing *PTEN*.

Penetrance of Cowden syndrome is age-dependent. Nearly all patients will develop mucocutaneous lesions by the third decade of life. The mutation spectrum of patients with Cowden syndrome and BRRS overlaps.

Clinical picture

Juvenile polyposis syndrome

The clinical diagnosis of JPS has been compartmentalised into one of three categories: i) juvenile polyposis of infancy; ii) juvenile polyposis coli (colonic involvement only); or iii) generalised juvenile polyposis [14]. Juvenile polyposis of infancy has an onset in the first two years of life and has a generally poor prognosis. These patients often present with recurrent gastrointestinal bleeding, diarrhoea, protein-losing enteropathy, intussusception, and/or rectal prolapse [14]. This condition has been associated with a contiguous gene deletion of *PTEN* and *BMPRIA* [15].

Polyposis

Juvenile polyposis coli and generalised juvenile polyposis represent variable expression of JPS. Most patients will have polyps by their second decade of life and may develop a few to hundreds of polyps over their lifetime. Patients may present with chronic or acute gastrointestinal bleeding, anaemia, prolapsed rectal polyps, abdominal pain, or diarrhoea [16]. Polyps occur throughout the gastrointestinal tract including the colon and rectum, stomach, and small bowel.

Malignancy risk

Patients with JPS have approximately a 50% lifetime risk of developing colorectal cancer with a range of 17-68% reported in the literature [17]. The mean age of colorectal cancer diagnosis for patients with JPS is 43 years [18]. Cancers also may develop in the stomach, duodenum, pancreas, and jejunum. The risk of gastric or duodenal cancer is 15-21% [18]. Neoplastic degeneration is more likely to occur in patients with the generalised form of polyposis compared with those with colorectal polyposis only [17]. The youngest reported cancer occurred in a 15-year-old but the majority of cases occur in the third and fourth decade of life.

Other manifestations

Congenital defects have also been associated with JPS including abnormalities of the heart and cranium, cleft palate, polydactyly, and malrotation of the gut. Most often, these defects occur in sporadic cases.

Peutz-Jeghers syndrome

Polyposis

Gastrointestinal hamartomatous polyps associated with a distinctive mucocutaneous pigmentation are the key clinical features of PJS. Approximately 88% of patients with PJS will develop polyps, which most commonly occur in the small bowel, colon, stomach, and rectum. In rare cases, polyps have also occurred in the renal pelvis, urinary bladder, lungs, and nares. Usually, the total number of polyps is less than 20 and individual polyps vary in size from a few millimeters to several centimeters. Symptoms usually develop by the second or third decade of life. The various clinical presentations of patients with gastrointestinal polyposis include obstruction, abdominal pain, gastrointestinal bleeding, polyp prolapse per anus, or recurrent small bowel intussusception.

Mucocutaneous pigmentation

The characteristic pigmentation of PJS is present in approximately 95% of cases and occurs most commonly on the vermillion border of the lips (94%), buccal mucosa (66%), hands (74%) and feet (62%), but has also been reported in the peri-orbital, peri-anal, and genital areas [19]. Typically these lesions present as small, dark brown or blue-brown macules in infancy and may fade in late adolescence.

Malignancy risk

Patients with PJS are also at increased risk of developing malignancies. A meta-analysis of 210 patients from six publications estimated a 93% lifetime risk of developing cancer [20]. The cancers with the most significantly increased risk are breast (54%), colon (39%), pancreas (36%), and stomach (29%). Rare cancers in the reproductive organs are also associated with PJS. Among women with this syndrome, sex-cord tumours with annular tubules of the ovary and adenoma malignum of the cervix have been reported. These tumours can cause irregular menstruation and precocious puberty. Men are at risk for testicular tumours of sex-cord and Sertoli-cell type that are associated with gynaecomastia and sexual precocity.

PTEN-hamartoma tumour syndrome

Cowden syndrome

Cowden syndrome is believed to occur in 1 in every 200,000 individuals, but this is likely an underestimate. It is characterised by multiple hamartomas which can affect derivatives of any of the three germ layers, mucocutaneous lesions, macrocephaly, and an increased risk of benign and malignant disease of the breast, thyroid, and endometrium [21]. Nearly all patients with Cowden syndrome have the mucocutaneous lesions (Figure 1), which include trichilemmomas, papillomatous papules,

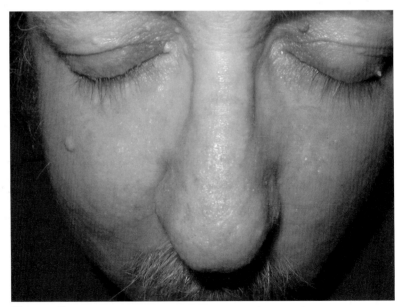

Figure 1. Cutaneous lesions found in Cowden syndrome.

and acral keratosis. Women have a 50% lifetime risk of developing breast cancer and a 5-10% lifetime risk of developing endometrial cancer. Fibrocystic disease of the breasts, uterine fibroids, and other genitourinary malformations are also prominent features of Cowden syndrome. Men and women with Cowden syndrome have a 10% lifetime risk of developing epithelial thyroid cancer, believed to be predominantly follicular histology. Thyroid nodules and goitre are also part of the disease spectrum. Hamartomatous polyps have been reported in patients with Cowden syndrome, although they have not been recognised as a major component of the condition. A few studies estimated that 60-90% of patients have diminutive colonic polyps distal to the hepatic flexure.

Bannayan-Riley-Ruvalcaba syndrome

BRRS is characterised by macrocephaly, developmental delay, lipomatosis, gastrointestinal hamartomatous polyps, haemangiomatosis, and pigmented macules on the glans penis in males. Initially, patients with BRRS were not thought to have an increased risk of malignancy, but currently it is believed that all patients with *PTEN* mutations carry the same malignancy risk as those with Cowden syndrome. Approximately half of the patients with BRRS will have hamartomatous polyps in the digestive tract, particularly in the ileum and colon. These polyps can cause intussusception and rectal bleeding but are not believed to increase the risk of colon cancer.

Proteus syndrome

The prominent features of Proteus syndrome are congenital malformations, hemihypertrophy, hamartomatous overgrowths, and epidermal nevi with a mosaic distribution [22]. The course of disease is progressive and the cases are sporadic. There is no known association of polyposis in patients with Proteus syndrome. Cancer or tumours have rarely been reported in patients with Proteus syndrome, particularly cystadenomas of the ovary, various testicular tumours, central nervous system tumours, and parotid monomorphic adenomas.

Diagnosis and surveillance

Juvenile polyposis syndrome

A clinical diagnosis of JPS is considered in patients with: i) more than five juvenile polyps of the colon or rectum; ii) juvenile polyps in other parts of the gastrointestinal tract; or iii) any number of juvenile polyps and a positive family history. All patients that satisfy these criteria should be offered genetic counselling and genetic testing.

Genetic testing

Genetic testing is available in the United States and Europe. Approximately 54% of cases will have a detectable mutation in *SMAD4* or *BMPR1A*. Once a mutation is identified in a proband, at-risk family members can be tested for the family-specific mutation. Approximately 75% of patients will have an affected parent. If one of the parents is affected, then testing should be offered to the siblings of the proband. Additionally, all children of the proband will have a 50% chance of inheriting the mutation and should be tested accordingly. After appropriate genetic counselling and informed consent, testing for at-risk family members may be performed during the teenage years.

Clinical surveillance

Colonoscopic surveillance for patients with JPS is recommended to begin at age 15 or earlier if symptoms develop. Full colonoscopy is warranted, as the right colon is also prone to developing polyps and cancer. If no polyps are identified, then repeat colonoscopy is recommended at three-year intervals. Any polyps should be removed endoscopically and sent for pathological examination. Repeat examination should be performed annually until no polyps are seen, at which time the screening interval should return to every three years. If dysplasia is identified or the polyp burden cannot be managed colonoscopically, colectomy is advocated. Other indications for surgery are discussed below.

Upper gastrointestinal surveillance should commence between age 15-25 or earlier if symptoms develop. Endoscopic management principles follow those as given for colonoscopy.

Peutz-Jeghers syndrome

A clinical diagnosis of PJS is based on the World Health Organization criteria: i) three or more histologically confirmed Peutz-Jeghers polyps; or ii) any number of Peutz-Jeghers polyps with a family history of PJS; or iii) characteristic, prominent, mucocutaneous pigmentation with a family history of PJS; or iv) any number of Peutz-Jeghers polyps and characteristic prominent, mucocutaneous pigmentation. It is recommended that genetic testing be offered to any patient with at least one Peutz-Jeghers polyp or mucocutaneous pigmentation.

Genetic testing

Testing is available in the United States and Europe. Sequencing and multiplex ligation-dependent probe amplification will identify mutations in 94% of patients who meet the diagnostic criteria. Once a mutation is identified in a proband, at-risk family members can be tested for this family-specific alteration. Approximately half of cases will have an affected parent. Parents of apparently isolated cases should be carefully evaluated for features of PJS. If one of the parents is affected, then testing should be offered to the siblings of the proband. Additionally, all children of the proband have a 50% risk of inheriting the mutation and should be tested accordingly. After appropriate genetic counselling and informed consent, testing for at-risk family members may be performed during childhood.

Clinical surveillance

Once a patient is diagnosed with PJS, regular surveillance is necessary. Although there have not been controlled studies documenting the efficacy of cancer surveillance in PJS, recommendations have been derived by published expert opinion. Due to the increased risk of malignancy in multiple organ systems, surveillance strategies are rather complex. The type and timing of specific tests are determined by the patient's age and sex. One proposed screening paradigm is summarised in Figure 2 overleaf.

Surveillance of small bowel polyposis has traditionally been difficult as the majority of mucosa is not easily accessible by endoscopy. Newer techniques such as capsule endoscopy and double-balloon enteroscopy have been employed to identify jejunal and ileal polyps.

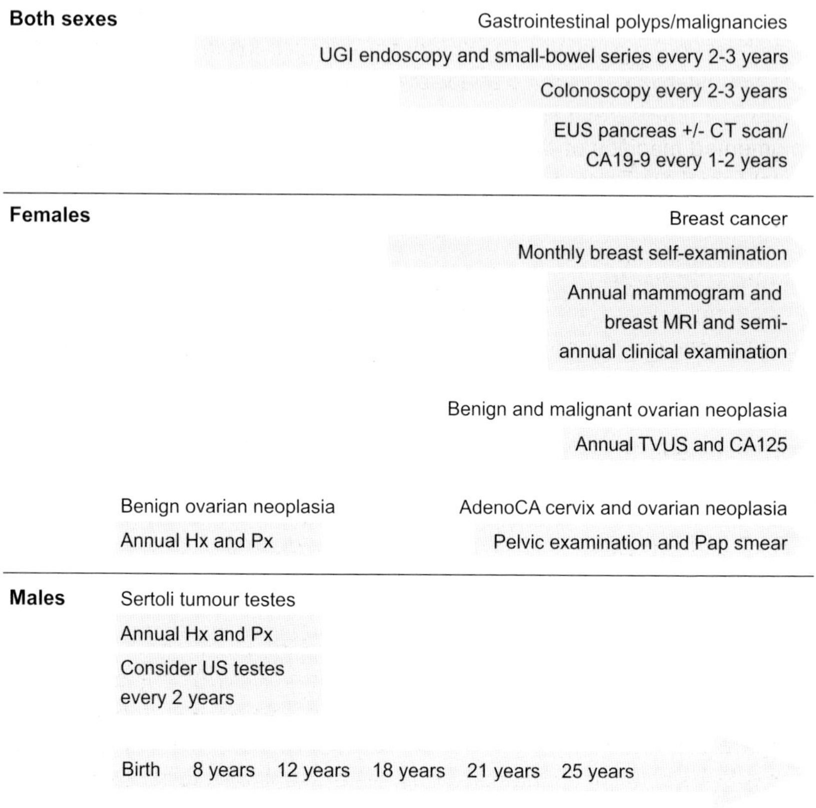

Both sexes		Gastrointestinal polyps/malignancies
		UGI endoscopy and small-bowel series every 2-3 years
		Colonoscopy every 2-3 years
		EUS pancreas +/- CT scan/ CA19-9 every 1-2 years
Females		Breast cancer
		Monthly breast self-examination
		Annual mammogram and breast MRI and semi-annual clinical examination
		Benign and malignant ovarian neoplasia
		Annual TVUS and CA125
	Benign ovarian neoplasia	AdenoCA cervix and ovarian neoplasia
	Annual Hx and Px	Pelvic examination and Pap smear
Males	Sertoli tumour testes	
	Annual Hx and Px	
	Consider US testes every 2 years	
	Birth 8 years 12 years 18 years 21 years 25 years	

Figure 2. Proposed screening paradigm for patients with PJS. Abbreviations: EUS=endoscopic ultrasound; Hx=history; Pap smear= Papanicolaou smear; Px=physical exam; TVUS=transvaginal ultrasound; UGI=upper gastrointestinal; US=ultrasound. *Reproduced with permission from the author* [23].

PTEN-hamartoma tumour syndrome

A PHTS diagnosis can be considered based on clinical findings, but a definitive, gene-based diagnosis can only be made upon identifying a germline *PTEN* mutation. The International Cowden Consortium has proposed operational clinical diagnostic criteria for Cowden syndrome, which are outlined in Table 1 [23]. Consensus diagnostic criteria for BRRS are not established, but a diagnosis is considered in patients with the key features of macrocephaly, hamartomatous colonic polyposis, lipomas, and pigmented macules of the glans penis. Diagnostic criteria have also been established for Proteus syndrome [22], but are not elaborated upon in this chapter.

Genetic testing

Genetic testing is available in the United States and Europe. Testing should include sequencing of all coding exons and flanking intronic regions, analysis for large deletions/rearrangements, and sequencing of the promoter. It is unclear how many cases are due to new mutation. Therefore, parents of gene-positive patients should be offered testing. All offspring of an affected individual have a 50% chance of inheriting the mutation. It is appropriate to offer testing to family members prior to the age of 18, since BRRS and Proteus syndrome can have onset in childhood.

Clinical surveillance

It is recommended that all patients with *PTEN* mutations follow the surveillance outlined for patients with Cowden syndrome (Table 2) [23]. Cancer surveillance is targeted to the breasts, thyroid, and endometrium. There are no specific recommendations for colon cancer or polyposis surveillance as there are no data about the true prevalence of colon cancer in Cowden syndrome. However, patients with BRRS should be monitored for complications caused by polyposis.

Clinical management

Juvenile polyposis syndrome

Due to the cancer risk, surgical intervention remains a crucial part of managing patients with JPS. Historically, some physicians had recommended prophylactic colectomy by age 20, but there is no evidence that this reduces cancer development compared to compliant surveillance protocols with polypectomy. Colectomy is warranted for the presence of cancer or dysplasia, or for patients with symptoms. Prophylactic

Table 1. Consensus criteria for Cowden syndrome.

An operational diagnosis of Cowden syndrome is made if an individual meets any one of the following criteria:

◆ Pathognomonic mucocutaneous lesions alone if there are:
  - six or more facial papules, of which three or more must be trichilemmoma; or
  - cutaneous facial papules and oral mucosal papillomatosis; or
  - oral mucosal papillomatosis and acral keratoses; or
  - six or more palmoplantar keratoses.
◆ Two or more major criteria.
◆ One major and at least three minor criteria.
◆ At least four minor criteria.

In a family in which one individual meets the diagnostic criteria for Cowden syndrome listed above, other relatives are considered to have a diagnosis of CS if they meet any of the following criteria:

◆ The pathognomonic criteria.
◆ Any one major criterion with or without minor criteria.
◆ Two minor criteria.
◆ History of Bannayan-Riley-Ruvalcaba syndrome.

Pathognomonic criteria: adult L'Hermitte-Duclos disease (LDD), mucocutaneous lesions, trichilemmomas (facial), acral keratoses, papillomatous lesions.

Major criteria: breast cancer, thyroid cancer (non-medullary), especially follicular, macrocephaly, endometrial carcinoma.

Minor criteria: other thyroid lesions (e.g. adenoma, multinodular goitre), mental retardation, gastrointestinal hamartomas, fibrocystic breast disease, lipomas, fibromas, genitourinary tumours, genitourinary malformation.

Table 2. Medical management for Cowden syndrome.

- Annual physical exam starting at age 18 years or five years younger than the earliest diagnosis of cancer in the family.
- Annual urinalysis. Consider annual urine cytololgy and renal ultrasound examination if there is a family history of renal cancer.
- Baseline thyroid ultrasound examination at age 18 years with annual follow-up.
- Annual dermatology examination.
- Baseline colonoscopy at age 50.

Specific surveillance for women:

- Monthly breast self-examination starting at age 18.
- Annual clinical breast examinations starting at age 25 years or 5-10 years earlier than the youngest diagnosis in the family.
- Annual mammogram and breast MRI starting at age 30-35 years or 5-10 years earlier than the youngest diagnosis in the family.
- Consideration of prophylactic mastectomy.
- Annual blind endometrial aspiration biopsies for premenopausal women starting at age 35-40 years or 5-10 years earlier than the youngest diagnosis in the family.
- Annual endometrial ultrasound examination for postmenopausal women.

colectomy should also be considered for patients whose polyp burden cannot be controlled endoscopically, for patients whose family history includes colorectal cancer, and for patients with poor compliance, which would result in an inability to perform timely surveillance.

Surgical options for colonic disease include colectomy with ileorectal anastomosis, or total proctocolectomy with an end ileostomy or formation of an ileoanal anastomosis. Creation of a permanent end ileostomy is generally not preferred by patients and is rarely used. Surgical decision-making is based on balancing the risks of developing symptoms or cancer within the remaining rectum after colectomy and ileorectal anastomosis versus the risks of a more extensive operation and potentially worse bowel function after a total proctocolectomy and ileal pouch-to-anal anastomosis. It is the author's preference (MFK) to leave the rectum in place and perform total abdominal colectomy with ileorectal anastomosis unless there is cancer in the rectum or symptoms are being caused by disease in the rectum. This operation avoids the potential complications of pelvic surgery and results in improved bowel function, an issue which is particularly important for younger patients.

A study done at the Cleveland Clinic evaluated the outcomes of patients using this approach [24]. Of the ten patients that underwent a rectum-preserving surgery, five of them eventually required a proctectomy within a median time of nine years (range 6-34 years). Interestingly, there was no correlation between the number of polyps in the rectum and the need for proctectomy. It is also important to note continued surveillance is still required regardless of the surgery performed since polyps may develop in the remaining rectum or ileal pouch [24].

Since the cancer risk is lower in the upper gastrointestinal tract compared with the colon, surgical intervention is based on symptoms, evidence of malignant change, or protein-losing gastropathy/enteropathy. Subtotal gastrectomy is usually the procedure of choice for disease in the stomach and segmental resection is performed for small bowel disease.

Peutz-Jeghers syndrome

Clinical management of PJS can be divided into prophylactic intervention and treatment of polyp-related complications. Similar to the surveillance guidelines, prophylactic interventions for lesions that are found during routine surveillance are based on recommendations by expert opinions rather than controlled studies. Asymptomatic gastric or colonic polyps greater than 1cm in size should be removed endoscopically. Similarly, rapidly growing small bowel polyps or those greater than 1-1.5cm should also be removed to decrease the potential development of complications. The most common complications requiring intervention are bleeding and intussusception. Slowly bleeding polyps causing anaemia may be managed endoscopically if able to be reached. An endoscopic approach combined with laparoscopy or laparotomy, which allows the surgeon to guide the endoscope, may be employed to reach the lesion of interest. Obstruction is managed surgically by laparoscopy or laparotomy with resection of the inciting polyp. Some authors favour complete removal of all polyps found in the gastrointestinal tract at the time of surgery to achieve a 'clean sweep'. In this situation, elimination of all polyps reduces the need for future surgery.

PTEN-hamartoma tumour syndrome

The central principle of management of individuals with PHTS entails making an accurate diagnosis and assessing individual cancer risk, leading to organ-specific clinical surveillance (above section).

When individuals with germline *PTEN* mutations are ascertained by Cowden syndrome or Cowden-like syndromes, it appears that gastrointestinal polyps are present but not a prominent feature. Whether Cowden-related polyps result in an increased risk of colorectal cancers is unknown and pends further research. Colon surveillance is not routinely recommended for such individuals beyond that for the general population, unless there happens to be colorectal cancer in the family. In BRRS, colonic polyposis may be prominent (see above), and is treated symptomatically.

Women with *PTEN* mutations may consider prophylactic mastectomy as a preventive measure. This surgery has been shown to reduce the risk of breast cancer by as much as 90% in other high-risk populations. Currently, no specific studies have evaluated the effectiveness of this surgery in patients with Cowden syndrome. Nonetheless, patients with Cowden syndrome often have bilateral benign breast disease, such as breast hamartomas, fibroadenomas and fibrocystic disease [23]. When these benign neoplasias and harmatomas are extensive, surveillance, even with breast MRI, might prove difficult. In such a situation, it may be reasonable to consider bilateral prophylactic mastectomies.

Chemoprevention with tamoxifen and raloxifene has been shown to reduce the risk of breast cancer in other high-risk populations. There is no direct evidence that this is effective therapy in women with Cowden syndrome. Additionally, tamoxifen has been shown to increase the risk of endometrial cancer in populations already at increased risk. Therefore, this intervention should be considered cautiously for patients with Cowden syndrome.

Unless the thyroid becomes difficult to screen, clinical surveillance of the thyroid should be sufficient. When an individual with PHTS develops epithelial thyroid carcinoma, at a minimum, a total thyroidectomy should be performed, even in T1 (stage 1) disease. This is because of the continued increased risk of developing a second primary cancer in any remnant tissue. Equally importantly, individuals with germline *PTEN* mutations scar excessively and a second operation would prove technically challenging Other than these two considerations, epithelial thyroid cancer in individuals with PHTS should be treated no differently from sporadic cases pending further data.

Although no formal studies exist, one genotype-phenotype study suggests that there is an increased risk of endometrial carcinoma and surveillance is recommended. In the absence of PHTS-related endometrial carcinoma treatment, once this cancer has developed, it should be treated no differently than in sporadic cases.

Often, managing the benign manifestations of Cowden syndrome proves equally challenging. There is little issue when these benign neoplasias and hamartomas are asymptomatic, and if this is true, then these lesions should not be removed. Although there are no formal studies, surgical resection of benign Cowden-related lesions usually results in recurrence of the lesions and scarring. When these benign neoplasias or hamartomas are threatening vital organs, cause severe pain or it is unclear if they are malignant, then surgical extirpation may be warranted.

The future

Despite the seemingly distinct presentations distinguishing each of these hamartomatous polyposis syndromes, making the correct diagnosis for these conditions can be challenging, as significant overlap exists. At least one study has noted that substantial discrepancies were identified in the histopathology of patients with at least one hyperplastic or hamartomatous polyp when re-reviewed by a dedicated gastrointestinal pathologist, and demonstrating the usefulness of molecular classification of the polyp conditions [8]. The availability of genetic testing for these conditions has improved our ability to accurately diagnose these patients. However, for a number of patients, e.g. JPS, the underlying genetic aetiology has not been identified. We also suspect that the hamartomatous polyposes as a group are genetically heterogeneous and so other susceptibility alleles, whether high or low penetrance, need to be sought.

In the future, the molecular or genetic classification of the hamartoma polyposis syndromes and conditions would not only serve the purpose for accurate diagnosis, but also for selection of therapy or prevention. For example, PTEN dysfunction leads to increased AKT and mTOR signalling (see above and Figure 3). Therefore, mTOR inhibitors may be considered

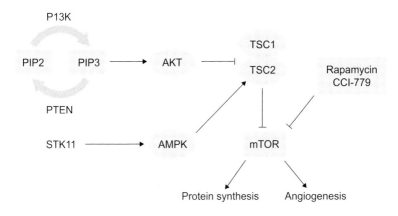

Figure 3. Signalling pathway for PTEN and STK11. Abbreviations: AKT=protein kinase B; AMPK=AMP-activated protein kinase; mTOR=mammalian target of rapamycin; PI3K=phosphoinositide-3 kinase; PIP2=phosphoinositol 4,5-bisphosphate; PIP3=phosphoinositol 3,4,5-trisphosphate; PTEN=phosphatase and tensin homologue, deleted on chromosome 10; STK11=serine-threonine protein kinase 11; TSC1=tuberous sclerosis 1 protein; TSC2=tuberous sclerosis 2 protein. *Reproduced with permission from the author* [23].

for those with germline *PTEN* abnormalities. The protein encoded by the PJS susceptibility gene, STK11/LKB1, is upstream of PTEN and negatively regulates the mTOR pathway, and so it may be reasonable to postulate that mTOR inhibition could be useful in this condition as well. The thiazolidinediones and statins have been shown, at least *in vitro*, to upregulate PTEN and in the future, may serve a therapeutic and/or preventative role. Similarly, BMP2 has been shown to stabilise PTEN protein and may play dual roles in PHTS and polyposes where the BMP pathway is involved.

Key points

♦ The hamartomatous polyposis syndromes are a rare group of autosomal dominant conditions characterised by the presence of hamartomatous polyps in the gastrointestinal tract.

♦ Juvenile polyposis syndrome is caused by mutations in *SMAD4*, *BMPR1A*, and *ENG1*. Patients with this condition are at increased risk of colonic and upper gastrointestinal tract cancers.

♦ The defining features of Peutz-Jeghers syndrome are mucocutaneous pigmentation, small bowel polyposis, and an increased risk of intestinal and extra-intestinal malignancy. Mutations in *STK11* cause this syndrome.

♦ The PTEN-hamartoma tumour syndrome is composed of Cowden syndrome, Bannayan-Riley-Ruvalcaba syndrome, and Proteus syndrome. Nearly half of patients with Bannayan-Riley-Ruvalcaba syndrome will have hamartomatous polyps.

♦ Each one of these syndromes has unique risks that require tailored medical management.

References

1. McColl I, Bussey HJ, Veale AM, Morson BC. Juvenile polyposis coli. *Proc R Soc Med* 1964; 57: 896-7.
2. Peutz J. A very peculiar familial polyposis of the mucous membrane of the digestive tract and the nasopharynx together with peculiar pigmentation of the skin and mucous membranes. *Ned Maandschr Geneesk* 1921; 10: 134.
3. Jeghers H, Mc KV, Katz KH. Generalized intestinal polyposis and melanin spots of the oral mucosa, lips and digits; a syndrome of diagnostic significance. *N Engl J Med* 1949; 241(25): 993, illust; passim.
4. Bannayan GA. Lipomatosis, angiomatosis, and macrencephalia. A previously undescribed congenital syndrome. *Arch Pathol* 1971; 92(1): 1-5.
5. Marsh DJ, Kum JB, Lunetta KL, *et al*. *PTEN* mutation spectrum and genotype-phenotype correlations in Bannayan-Riley-Ruvalcaba syndrome suggest a single entity with Cowden syndrome. *Hum Mol Genet* 1999; 8(8): 1461-72.
6. Schwartz RA. Basal-cell-nevus syndrome and gastrointestinal polyposis. *N Engl J Med* 1978; 299(1): 49.
7. Jaeger EE, Woodford-Richens KL, Lockett M, *et al*. An ancestral Ashkenazi haplotype at the *HMPS/CRAC1* locus on 15q13-q14 is associated with hereditary mixed polyposis syndrome. *Am J Hum Genet* 2003; 72(5): 1261-7.
8. Sweet K, Willis J, Zhou XP, *et al*. Molecular classification of patients with unexplained hamartomatous and hyperplastic polyposis. *JAMA* 2005; 294(19): 2465-73.
9. Sayed MG, Ahmed AF, Ringold JR, *et al*. Germline *SMAD4* or *BMPR1A* mutations and phenotype of juvenile polyposis. *Ann Surg Oncol* 2002; 9(9): 901-6.
10. Eng C, Ji H. Molecular classification of the inherited hamartoma polyposis syndromes: clearing the muddied waters. *Am J Hum Genet* 1998; 62(5): 1020-2.
11. Howe JR, Sayed MG, Ahmed AF, *et al*. The prevalence of *MADH4* and *BMPR1A* mutations in juvenile polyposis and absence of *BMPR2*, *BMPR1B*, and *ACVR1* mutations. *J Med Genet* 2004; 41(7): 484-91.
12. Friedl W, Uhlhaas S, Schulmann K, *et al*. Juvenile polyposis: massive gastric polyposis is more common in *MADH4* mutation carriers than in *BMPR1A* mutation carriers. *Hum Genet* 2002; 111(1): 108-11.
13. Gallione CJ, Repetto GM, Legius E, *et al*. A combined syndrome of juvenile polyposis and hereditary haemorrhagic telangiectasia associated with mutations in *MADH4* (*SMAD4*). *Lancet* 2004; 363(9412): 852-9.
14. Sachatello CR, Hahn IS, Carrington CB. Juvenile gastrointestinal polyposis in a female infant: report of a case and review of the literature of a recently recognized syndrome. *Surgery* 1974; 75(1): 107-14.
15. Delnatte C, Sanlaville D, Mougenot JF, *et al*. Contiguous gene deletion within chromosome arm 10q is associated with juvenile polyposis of infancy, reflecting co-operation between the *BMPR1A* and *PTEN* tumor-suppressor genes. *Am J Hum Genet* 2006; 78(6): 1066-74.
16. Merg A, Howe JR. Genetic conditions associated with intestinal juvenile polyps. *Am J Med Genet C Semin Med Genet* 2004; 129(1): 44-55.

17. Agnifili A, Verzaro R, Gola P, *et al.* Juvenile polyposis: case report and assessment of the neoplastic risk in 271 patients reported in the literature. *Dig Surg* 1999; 16(2): 161-6.

18. Brosens LA, van Hattem A, Hylind LM, *et al.* Risk of colorectal cancer in juvenile polyposis. *Gut* 2007; 56(7): 965-7.

19. Giardiello FM, Trimbath JD. Peutz-Jeghers syndrome and management recommendations. *Clin Gastroenterol Hepatol* 2006; 4(4): 408-15.

20. Giardiello FM, Brensinger JD, Tersmette AC, *et al.* Very high risk of cancer in familial Peutz-Jeghers syndrome. *Gastroenterology* 2000; 119(6): 1447-53.

21. Eng C. Will the real Cowden syndrome please stand up: revised diagnostic criteria. *J Med Genet* 2000; 37(11): 828-30.

22. Biesecker LG, Happle R, Mulliken JB, *et al.* Proteus syndrome: diagnostic criteria, differential diagnosis, and patient evaluation. *Am J Med Genet* 1999; 84(5): 389-95.

23. Zbuk KM, Eng C. Hamartomatous polyposis syndromes. *Nat Clin Pract Gastroenterol Hepatol* 2007; 4(9): 492-502.

24. Oncel M, Church JM, Remzi FH, Fazio VW. Colonic surgery in patients with juvenile polyposis syndrome: a case series. *Dis Colon Rectum* 2005; 48(1): 49-55; discussion -6.

Chapter 14

The future structure of care: cancer genetics

Andrew Beggs MRCS
Research Registrar in Colorectal Surgery
Mayday University Hospital, London and
Honorary Research Fellow in Cancer Genetics
St George's, University of London, UK

Shirley Hodgson FRCP DM
Professor of Cancer Genetics
St George's, University of London
and Honorary Consultant
St George's Hospital, London, UK

Background

With the rapid advance in molecular diagnostic technologies and the recognition of the value of a well taken family history as well as counselling, contacting and testing affected relatives, clinicians with a specialist interest in cancer genetics should now play a vital role as part of the multi-disciplinary team in the care of the patient with cancer.

Initially, the specialty of cancer genetics started in the late 1980s as 'family history' clinics to which patients thought to be at increased risk of cancer because of a strong family history of cancer were referred for assessment [1]. With the introduction of reproducible molecular genetic tests for inherited cancer susceptibility, the role of the cancer genetics clinic expanded to include identifying patients at risk, carrying out diagnostic testing and offering screening and appropriate genetic testing to their relatives based on risk assessment.

Immunohistochemical staining of colorectal cancers for features of Lynch syndrome and the use of hormone receptor and HER2 staining of breast cancers to identify individuals at increased risk of having a germline mutation in *BRCA1*, should become a routine part of the assessment of all cancers in the general population.

Future developments in the role of cancer genetics in the care that can be offered to patients include the setting up of genetic risk assessment clinics in primary and secondary care, risk prediction based on DNA single nucleotide polymorphism (SNP) analysis, with targeting of screening to those individuals in the highest percentiles of risk, and non-invasive molecular screening. The tailoring of chemotherapeutic agents based on gene expression profiles and genotypes is also an emerging area, with a potential to revolutionise therapy.

Family history and risk assessment

A well taken, comprehensive family history is still the most helpful [2] initial form of genetic risk assessment, and will be for the foreseeable future. Consensus guidelines such as the Amsterdam [3] and Bethseda [4] guidelines for hereditary non-polyposis colonic cancer (HNPCC) have allowed clinicians to identify with a good degree of accuracy the types of family in which genetic testing of an affected family member is likely to identify a germline mutation in a cancer susceptibility gene such as those causing Lynch syndrome. This allows triage and risk stratification in the community setting and, if appropriate, referral onwards for further genetic counselling.

Service models

The Kenilworth consensus guidelines (2001) [5] were proposed as a model for future cancer genetics services. Several pilot centres were set up across the UK, whereby different service models were assessed and applied to local needs. The aims of the Kenilworth model are that patients should be counselled with consistent and correct information, a standardised risk assessment carried out, and individuals managed according to the level of risk based on the risk assessment.

Currently, most cancer genetics clinics in the UK are run in Regional Genetics Centres as part of the general genetics service, and these may oversee several clinics at hospitals within the region they serve. Given the potential volume of referrals a cancer genetics clinic may receive, there have been various models for obtaining greater coverage and ascertaining more at-risk individuals. The usual model involves a central genetics clinic, usually in a teaching hospital, overseeing the provision of local services at the district general hospital level, staffed by a clinical geneticist and genetics counsellor. More specialised clinics are carried out at the central clinic. High-risk families may then be referred to the Regional Genetics Service.

Another model is a nurse-led clinic in primary care, whereby a nurse trained in cancer genetics and genetic counselling carries out clinics in primary care practices to categorise patients into low, medium and high risk. Low-risk patients can be reassured and discharged, whereas those at medium and high risk can be referred on to the central genetics clinic where surveillance can be arranged and monitored, and appropriate molecular diagnostic testing and counselling can be carried out.

Telephone assessment services can be used, with patients being assessed and counselled over the telephone. These could be run by the central cancer genetics clinics. A drawback of this approach, however, is in the patient assessed as high risk where patients' questions regarding their assessment and treatment may not be satisfactorily resolved via telephone, and onward referral to the genetics centre is clearly indicated. Language barriers may also be more of a problem than in face-to-face clinics with interpreters.

As part of a future model of care, one ideal would be to have either a nurse counsellor or clinical geneticist available in every cancer clinic in each hospital in a network. Each patient could be assessed and appropriately counselled. Those who need onward referral for testing for themselves and their family could be referred on to a central genetics clinic. This would allow care to be implemented at the local level but with the support and facilities of a centralised service.

Polymorphisms and risk profiles

The Human Genome Project [6], started in 1990 and completed in 2003, was a collaborative project between the National Institutes of Health in the USA and the Wellcome Trust in the UK. It was designed to sequence, map and identify the entire set of genes in human DNA (approximately 20,000-25,000), as well as to identify single nucleotide polymorphisms (SNP) in human DNA.

SNPs (Figure 1) are single amino acid alterations in the sequence of a human gene. They are common, and occur at least every 100-300 bases along the human genome, in both coding and non-coding regions. For a variation to be considered an SNP, it must occur in approximately 1% of the population.

The majority of SNPs are thought to have no effect on gene function; however, a small subset can cause a pathological change in the protein product such that it may confer an increased risk of disease. SNPs have been postulated to be responsible for the differences in progress of disease and response to treatment in affected patients.

Complementary to this, the International HapMap project [7] has been set up to develop a haplotype map of the human genome, using a reference set of subjects from various ethnic groups around the world. In the context of SNPs, a haplotype is a set of SNPs that are associated, and knowledge of these can be used to investigate the genetics behind common diseases, using SNP association studies.

Using the model of colorectal cancer, twin studies have shown that although the hereditable component of colorectal cancer susceptibility is approximately 30% [8], mutations in the high risk, 'classical' genes such as APC, the mismatch repair genes (MMR), MYH and others only account for 5% of this risk.

The remaining risk is thought to be due to SNPs and recent research in this area has concentrated on genome-wide scans for SNPs in large populations of colorectal cancer cases and controls to ascertain whether certain SNPs confer an increased risk of disease. Variation at 8q24 has

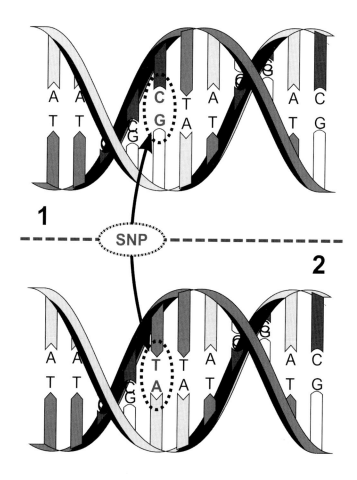

Figure 1. Diagram of single nucleotide polymorphism. *This diagram is reproduced under the Creative Commons Licence.* http://creativecommons.org/licenses/by/2.5/.

been identified as having a potential association with colorectal cancer in a recent study [9]. Further genome-wide studies are on-going with the expectation that other SNPs conferring an increased risk of disease will be found. This may allow individuals to be typed for a panel of SNPs, which individually may only confer a relative risk of 1.2-1.3 but collectively could allow a small proportion of individuals at a more substantial increased risk to be identified and targeted for increased surveillance.

The National Study of Colorectal Cancer Genetics (NSCCG) [10] recruits colorectal cancer patients and their partners as controls, with the aim of building up a library of 20,000 case-control pairs to aid in SNP discovery. As the study was carried out in the UK, its results may only be applicable to the UK population. With rapid advances in sequencing technology more pathogenic SNP variants will undoubtedly be identified. With this information available, it may be possible to produce a risk profile for a patient in terms of increased or decreased susceptibility to certain diseases.

As a consequence of the availability of SNP data, as well as sensitive and rapid DNA extraction methods, several commercial companies have been set up in order to use the SNP data to ascertain a risk profile based on the subject's DNA. Typically, a saliva sample containing cheek cells is obtained, and the sample analysed using a DNA-based microarray (such as the Illumina BeadArray®) designed for screening SNPs. The gene array uses an array of DNA probes tailored to specific SNPs and fluorescent probes that are hybridised with complementary DNA (cDNA) assembled from the subject's DNA. The gene array is scanned with a laser demonstrating fluorescence at regions where the SNP has been detected. This is then analysed by computer, allowing a rapid map of SNPs across the subject's whole genome to be built up. This allows rapid processing of a sample, but is based on a specific, fixed set of SNPs and is dependent upon the SNPs chosen for accuracy and validity of the result.

The companies currently offering this service only offer it via the internet, without face-to-face contact. They do not offer formal assessment, counselling and explanation of the results to the patient. Therefore, a patient may possess a SNP that only confers a very slightly increased risk of disease, but as the counselling and support systems that are in place in a genetics clinic do not exist in this setting, this kind of result may cause unnecessary worry for the patient, may not take into account all factors in predicting risk and could conversely lead to false reassurance and risk-taking behaviour.

Our knowledge of how SNPs affect disease progress is still in a very early stage. When understanding of how SNPs relate to total risk has expanded it may be possible to offer a risk prediction service as part of a genetics service. Patients may possess only one or two polymorphisms giving a very slightly increased risk and could be categorised as low risk, whereas patients who possess many pathogenic polymorphisms have a much increased lifetime risk and consequently a need for more regular screening. It is difficult to know who should be offered this kind of service. Enrolling all adults would overwhelm current facilities and also raises questions about cost-effectiveness issues, given the enormous resources required, in terms of laboratory facilities, data handling and counselling.

Currently, SNP risk profiling is an immature technology, and needs further research both on identifying pathogenic SNPs and an analysis of the cost-effectiveness of applying it to the entire population. Despite this, it has promise as an emerging technology and may well form a key part of cancer genetics clinics in the future.

Non-invasive molecular screening

Recent models of care in colorectal cancer have focused on population screening. The National Health Service (NHS) has instituted the National Bowel Cancer Screening Programme, based on a pilot study [11], using faecal occult blood testing (FOBT) kits to identify patients at risk of bowel cancer, and sending patients with positive FOBT either for colonoscopy or virtual colonoscopy. Since FOBT positivity is unlikely with adenomas, and tends to be seen only in the presence of a carcinoma, increased sensitivity could be developed using the detection of oncogenes in the faeces.

Family members of an affected proband identified as being at higher risk of colorectal cancer in the cancer genetics clinic or patients with at least one first-degree relative with bowel cancer are usually recommended to have regular surveillance colonoscopy based on the British Society of Gastroenterology [12] guidelines.

Colonoscopy allows total visualisation of the colon and identification and biopsy of very small lesions; however, it carries a risk of perforation estimated at 1:769 and therefore may not be suitable as a regular screening tool. The preparation that patients undergo for colonoscopy is unpleasant and may lead to reluctance to undergo regular colonoscopy.

Interest has been raised in the potential of faecal DNA markers for colorectal cancer, as this may allow a non-invasive method of screening at-risk relatives who present to cancer genetics clinics or in the general outpatient setting.

Potential molecular markers that have recently been identified include the hypermethylated secreted frizzled-related protein 2 (*SFRP2*) [13], *CDKN2A*, *MGMT*, and *MLH1* genes [14]. They are comparable to faecal occult blood testing in their sensitivity and specificity and have the potential to increase in their accuracy as improved assays are developed. Also, it has been shown that the presence of these markers increase in frequency as the histological stage of the adenoma progresses.

As more research is done into the earliest molecular changes in colorectal adenomas, more potential markers may be found. If the accuracy of testing improves, this may allow implementation of non-invasive, stool-based tests for screening patients in colorectal clinics who would normally have a colonoscopy. Patients who test positive using faecal DNA markers could then be sent for colonoscopy.

Undoubtedly, successful research in this area could stimulate similar tests for other inherited malignancies requiring screening. Early work has studied cytokeratin-19 mRNA levels in peripheral blood [15] of patients with early stage breast cancer, and as further markers are identified, patients with a family history of breast cancer needing screening may benefit from new methods of molecular screening, obviating the need for radiological screening and the potential risk from ionising radiation.

In conclusion, molecular screening of at-risk populations shows promise in screening families at risk of inherited malignancy. However, in order to maximise its effectiveness, it will inevitably need to be integrated with cancer genetics clinics in order to provide a safe, reproducible and reliable service.

Genomic oncology: the targeting of therapy

There has been much research recently in the field of tailoring chemotherapeutic agents to a patient's genetic expression profile. An example is the use of 5-fluorouracil (5-FU) chemotherapy in colorectal cancer. A proportion of patients with colorectal cancer may not have a therapeutic response to 5-FU. Alternative chemotherapeutic agents exist such as irinotecan and oxaliplatin that may be of benefit in these patients. A recent study [16] has shown that gene expression profiling is of use in predicting the response to chemotherapy in colon cancer cell lines and may be of use in predicting response in patients.

There are other examples where knowledge of the genotype influences patient management. In patients with breast cancer, poly(ADP-ribose) polymerase (PARP), an enzyme responsible for facilitating DNA damage repair has been identified as a therapeutic target for chemotherapeutic agents, as inhibition of PARP potentiates the activity of DNA-damaging chemotherapeutic agents [17]. As a consequence of this research it has been discovered that patients who possess *BRCA* mutations may be more susceptible to PARP inhibitors, several of which are currently undergoing phase 2 clinical trials.

Lynch syndrome which by definition is a mutation in the mismatch repair (MMR) enzyme system has been shown to alter the sensitivity of colorectal cancer cells to chemotherapeutic agents, with considerable evidence for resistance to the widely used 5-FU [18].

In conclusion, knowledge of the genotype of the patient is vital for oncological therapy, and as our knowledge of the pathway of tumourigenesis expands, it may be possible to further target agents based on a patient's pharmacogenomic profile.

Pre-implantation genetic diagnosis

Pre-implanatation genetic diagnosis (PGD) is a recently described technique whereby a couple in which one partner carries a disease-causing mutation can undergo screening of their embryos to ascertain whether the mutation is present [19] (Figure 2).

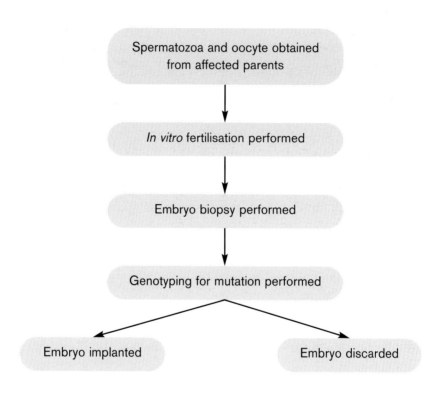

Figure 2. The process of pre-implantation genetic diagnosis.

PGD utilises embryos obtained via *in vitro* fertilisation. DNA is typically obtained at the earliest stage of fertilisation, usually around six days. Several techniques are used to obtain DNA, including blastomere biopsy, and less frequently, polar body removal. Genotyping is performed on a single extracted cell.

Mutations have been successfully screened for parents with familial adenomatous polyposis (*APC*), Li-Fraumeni syndrome (*TP53*), *BRCA1/2* mutations, retinoblastoma (*RB1*), multiple endocrine neoplasia Type 2A (*RET*), Fanconi anaemia (*FANCA*) and several other disorders [19, 20]. Unfortunately even with successful screening and elimination of embryos with the disease-carrying mutation, the successful implantation rate is very low. There are also significant dangers to the mother during the egg retrieval process, such as ovarian hyper-stimulation syndrome.

Use of PGD also raises several important ethical issues. Several of the conditions mentioned above either have low penetrance, or do not fully express the phenotype until the affected proband reaches adulthood, for example, in women with *BRCA1/2* mutations. Another example is probands with FAP who with colectomy and surveillance can have a very good life expectancy. Both of these cases raise the question of whether it is ethical to discard embryos carrying these mutations as they may well have a good quality of life for many years. In addition, treatment and prophylaxis in these conditions is likely to have improved in 20-30 years time.

As PGD technology evolves and our knowledge of disease-causing loci enlarges, it may become possible to screen for many mutations and genetic variants, which may alter disease susceptibility to variable degrees, raising the possibility of 'designer babies', as widely discussed recently in the press.

The future

The future path of cancer genetics is both exciting and uncertain. Our knowledge of the effect of genes on disease susceptibility has expanded exponentially in the last ten years, and thanks to new technologies such as DNA microarrays, multiplex ligation-dependent probe amplification (MLPA) and rapid sequencing, genetic analysis is becoming increasingly cost-effective and reliable.

As always, the entrepreneurial spirit has led to early adopters of these technologies making them available to the public, perhaps without full consideration of their implications and costs. Clinicians with a specific interest in cancer genetics and specialist cancer genetics clinics are well placed to be at the forefront of this 'genetic information revolution', and will further enhance the care of the cancer patient.

Key points

♦ Cancer genetics clinics remain the mainstay for identification of at-risk subjects.

♦ Nurse-led clinics may enable triage of patients into a central genetics service.

♦ The most highly penetrant susceptibility genes are *APC*, the *MMR* genes, *MYH* and other genes causing rarer cancer predisposing conditions.

♦ Single nucleotide polymorphisms (SNPs) are not currently very predictive of disease but may become increasingly important in risk stratification.

♦ Faecal DNA screening may have the potential to identify at-risk patients in large populations.

♦ Consideration of the genotype is important in tailoring therapy to specific patient groups (i.e. Lynch syndrome and 5-FU chemotherapy).

♦ Pre-implantation genetic diagnosis remains a controversial technology but may be useful in families with serious gene mutations.

References

1. Julian-Reynier C, Eisinger F, Chabal F, *et al*. Cancer genetics clinics: target population and consultees' expectations. *Eur J Cancer* 1996; 32A: 398-403.
2. Kelly KM, Sweet K. In search of a familial cancer risk assessment tool. *Clin Genet* 2007; 71: 76-83.

3.   Vasen HF, Watson P, Mecklin JP, *et al.* New clinical criteria for hereditary nonpolyposis colorectal cancer (HNPCC, Lynch syndrome) proposed by the International Collaborative group on HNPCC. *Gastroenterology* 1999; 116: 1453-6.

4.   Rodriguez-Bigas MA, Boland CR, Hamilton SR, *et al.* A National Cancer Institute Workshop on Hereditary Nonpolyposis Colorectal Cancer Syndrome: meeting highlights and Bethesda guidelines. *J Natl Cancer Inst* 1997; 89: 1758-62.

5.   Eeles R, Purland G, Maher J, *et al.* Delivering cancer genetics services - new ways of working. *Fam Cancer* 2007; 6: 163-7.

6.   Lander ES, Linton LM, Birren B, *et al.* Initial sequencing and analysis of the human genome. *Nature* 2001; 409: 860-921.

7.   Frazer KA, Ballinger DG, Cox DR, *et al.* A second generation human haplotype map of over 3.1 million SNPs. *Nature* 2007; 449: 851-61.

8.   Lichtenstein P, Holm NV, Verkasalo PK, *et al.* Environmental and heritable factors in the causation of cancer - analyses of cohorts of twins from Sweden, Denmark, and Finland. *N Engl J Med* 2000; 343: 78-85.

9.   Tomlinson I, Webb E, Carvajal-Carmona L, *et al.* A genome-wide association scan of tag SNPs identifies a susceptibility variant for colorectal cancer at 8q24.21. *Nat Genet* 2007; 39: 984-8.

10.   Penegar S, Wood W, Lubbe S, *et al.* National Study of Colorectal Cancer Genetics. *Br J Cancer* 2007; 97: 1305-9.

11.   Weller D, Coleman D, Robertson R, *et al.* The UK colorectal cancer screening pilot: results of the second round of screening in England. *Br J Cancer* 2007; 97: 1601-5.

12.   Dunlop MG. Guidance on large bowel surveillance for people with two first degree relatives with colorectal cancer or one first degree relative diagnosed with colorectal cancer under 45 years. *Gut* 2002; 51 Suppl 5: V17-20.

13.   Wang DR, Tang D. Hypermethylated *SFRP2* gene in fecal DNA is a high potential biomarker for colorectal cancer noninvasive screening. *World J Gastroenterol* 2008; 14: 524-31.

14.   Petko Z, Ghiassi M, Shuber A, *et al.* Aberrantly methylated *CDKN2A*, *MGMT*, and *MLH1* in colon polyps and in fecal DNA from patients with colorectal polyps. *Clin Cancer Res* 2005; 11: 1203-9.

15.   Ignatiadis M, Perraki M, Apostolaki S, *et al.* Molecular detection and prognostic value of circulating cytokeratin-19 messenger RNA-positive and HER2 messenger RNA-positive cells in the peripheral blood of women with early-stage breast cancer. *Clin Breast Cancer* 2007; 7: 883-9.

16.   Mariadason JM, Arango D, Shi Q, *et al.* Gene expression profiling-based prediction of response of colon carcinoma cells to 5-fluorouracil and camptothecin. *Cancer Res* 2003; 63: 8791-812.

17.   Ratnam K, Low JA. Current development of clinical inhibitors of poly(ADP-ribose) polymerase in oncology. *Clin Cancer Res* 2007; 13: 1383-8.

18.   Jover R, Zapater P, Castells A, *et al.* Mismatch repair status in the prediction of benefit from adjuvant fluorouracil chemotherapy in colorectal cancer. *Gut* 2006; 55: 848-55.

19.   Offit K, Kohut K, Clagett B, *et al.* Cancer genetic testing and assisted reproduction. *J Clin Oncol* 2006; 24: 4775-82.

20.   Spits C, De Rycke M, Van Ranst N, *et al.* Preimplantation genetic diagnosis for cancer predisposition syndromes. *Prenat Diagn* 2007; 27: 447-56.